CONNECTING GENDER AND AGEING

A Sociological Approach

Edited by
Sara Arber and Jay Ginn

Open University Press
Buckingham · Philadelphia

Open University Press
Celtic Court
22 Ballmoor
Buckingham
MK18 1XW

and
1900 Frost Road, Suite 101
Bristol, PA 19007, USA

First Published 1995
Reprinted 2002
Copyright © The Editors and Contributors, 1995

A catalogue record of this book is available from the British Library

ISBN 0 335 19471 0 (hb)   0 335 19470 2 (pb)

Library of Congress Cataloging-in-Publication Data

Connecting gender and ageing: a sociological approach/edited by
  Sara Arber and Jay Ginn.
      p.   cm.
    includes bibliographical references and index.
    ISBN 0-335-19471-0. – ISBN 0-335-19470-2 (pbk.)
    1. Aged-Attitudes. 2. Man-woman relationships. I. Arber, Sara,
  1949–   .II. Ginn, Jay.
  HQ1061.C646 1995
  305.26 – dc20   95–14729
                                                            CIP

100486(119 T

Typeset by Type Study, Scarborough
Printed in Great Britain by Marston Lindsay Ross International Ltd, Oxford

CONTENTS

LIST OF FIGURES AND TABLES

Figures

Tables

NOTES ON CONTRIBUTORS

Sara Arber is Professor of Sociology at the University of Surrey. She is co-author of *Gender and Later Life: A Sociological Analysis of Resources and Constraints* (1991, Sage) and co-editor of *Women and Working Lives* (1991, Macmillan) and *Ageing, Independence and the Life Course* (1993, Jessica Kingsley). Her current research is on older women's participation in paid employment and inequalities in women's health.

Janet Askham is a sociologist whose research career has spanned major life course issues, from marriage and fertility to mental and physical frailty in old age. Current research includes the marital relationships and financial circumstances of older people, and service issues, such as health promotion, services for dementia sufferers and accident prevention. She teaches the sociology of ageing at King's College London, where she is Deputy Director of the Age Concern Institute of Gerontology.

Miriam Bernard is Director of the MA/Diploma in Gerontology, Department of Applied Social Studies, Keele University. She has researched a range of issues relating to older people, and is working on an ESRC-funded project on older people and family life. She co-edited *Women Come of Age – Perspectives on the Lives of Older Women* (1993) and is writing a book on self-health care (Open University Press). She is an Executive Member of the British Society of Gerontology, and Chair of the North Staffordshire Association of Carers.

Errollyn Bruce is currently working as a community support worker with the Bradford Dementia Group, developing a support programme for family carers and investigating the support needs of so-called 'hidden carers'. She previously worked as a researcher with Hilary Rose, at the University of Bradford, on a project on caring among elderly couples.

Mike Bury was appointed Lecturer in Sociology at Bedford College, University of London in 1979. He was appointed to a University of London Chair in Sociology at Royal Holloway in 1991. Professor Bury is responsible for the MSc in Medical Sociology at Royal Holloway. His research interests are in the fields of ageing, disability and chronic illness, and mental health and cultural aspects of illness. He has published widely in these fields.

Lori D. Campbell is a doctoral candidate in the Department of Family Studies, and research assistant in the Gerontology Research Centre, University of Guelph, Ontario, Canada. She received her BA and MA in Sociology from the University of Western Ontario, London, Canada. Her research interests include men providing care to elderly relatives, singlehood in mid- and later life, and adult sibling ties.

Jay Ginn is a researcher at the National Institute for Social Work and was previously a Research Fellow in the Department of Sociology, University of Surrey. She has numerous publications on gender and ageing arising from research on gender inequality in older people's income and mid-life women's employment. She co-authored *Gender and Later Life: A Sociological Analysis of Resources and Constraints* (1991, Sage).

Doris Ingrisch is a Lecturer in the Department of History, University of Vienna, Austria and a freelance researcher. Her research interests are in women's history, ageing and gender, biography and connecting history and sociology. Her recent publications include *Research on Ageing in Austria, 1980–85* (Vienna, 1994) for the Ministry of Science and Research. She is researching 'Academics in exile: Intellectual culture and identity of exiled women and men'.

Catherine Itzin is an Inspector in the Social Services Inspectorate, Department of Health, and Honorary Research Fellow, Department of Applied Social Studies, University of Bradford. Dr Itzin is co-author of *I Don't Feel Old: Understanding the Experience of Later Life* (with P. Thompson and M. Abendstern, 1991); *Age Barriers at Work: Maximising the Potential of Mature and Older People* (with C. Phillipson, 1993) and *Gender, Culture and Organisational Change: Putting Theory into Practice* (with J. Newman, 1995).

Anne Martin Matthews is a Professor in the Department of Family Studies and Director of the Gerontology Research Centre, University of Guelph, Ontario, Canada. She is author of *Widowhood in Later Life* (1991, Butterworths) and publications on informal and formal support of the elderly, ageing in rural environments, and gender and ageing. Her current research involves the interface of work and family responsibilities.

Julie McMullin is a PhD candidate in Sociology at the University of Toronto and a researcher for the Centre for Studies of Aging, University of Toronto, and the Interdisciplinary Group on Aging, University of Western Ontario, Canada. Her published work has focused on older childless individuals. Her doctorate involves theoretical and empirical assessments of class, gender, and age bases of social inequality.

Chris Phillipson is Professor of Applied Social Studies and Social Gerontology at the University of Keele. He has published widely in the field of ageing studies and recently co-authored *Elder Abuse in Perspective* (Open University Press). He is preparing a book on theoretical perspectives in gerontology (Sage) and is working on a major ESRC-funded project on family and kinship patterns of older people.

Hilary Rose has taught at the University of Bradford since 1975. Professor Rose is currently an Honorary Fellow at the Social Science Research Unit, Institute of Education, London. In addition to researching on feminist issues in social policy she also contributes to feminist science studies. Her most recent book is *Love, Power and Knowledge: Towards a Feminist Transformation of the Sciences* (1994, Polity).

Anne Scott is a former mathematician with degrees from Cambridge and Warwick universities. She worked as a teacher and computer programmer before becoming interested in social research. She has previously researched disabled young people, infant feeding, and the epidemiology of dementia. In 1993 she joined the Centre for Social Policy Research and Development, University of Wales, Bangor, where she is investigating the support networks of elderly people with G. Clare Wenger.

Julie Skucha is currently studying full time for a doctorate at Wolverhampton University and teaching Women's Studies and Sociology part time. Her research is on mature female graduates' entry into the labour market. Prior to this, she conducted research on preretirement education for women in part time employment.

G. Clare Wenger is Professor of Social Gerontology at the University of Wales, Bangor, where she is co-director of the Centre for Social Policy Research and Development. Since 1978, she has been responsible for a longitudinal study of ageing focusing on support networks. She has published widely, and her latest book is *Support Networks of Older People: A Guide for Practitioners* (1994).

Terri Whittaker lectures in Ageing and Community Care at the University of Liverpool. She is a qualified social worker with experience in older people's services both as a practitioner and researcher. Her research interests include community care and inequalities in welfare, especially their effect on older people and their carers. She is currently writing a book on elder abuse based on research in two social service departments.

Gail Wilson is Lecturer in Social Policy and Ageing at the London School of Economics. She has worked on the distribution of resources within households and the evaluation of community care services for older people, and is currently involved in research on aspects of advanced ageing, elder abuse, ageing across Europe and interprofessional issues in the management of community services. She is co-editor (with J. Brannen) of *Give and Take in Families* (1987, Allen and Unwin).

PREFACE

There is growing interest in the fact that western societies are ageing and that women predominate in later life, yet the way gender and ageing interact has so far been neglected by feminist researchers and sociologists. This book seeks to redress this neglect and challenge the assumption that gender can be treated as static over the life course, highlighting the different social effects of ageing on women's and men's roles, relationships and identity.

Most of the chapters were originally presented at an international symposium on gender and ageing held at the University of Surrey in July 1994. The symposium stimulated a great deal of lively discussion, as well as resulting in the establishment of warm friendships and fruitful working relationships. We are grateful to all the participants at the symposium for their constructive and insightful comments, and to Linda Bates for her superb administrative arrangements.

The preparation of this volume has been a creative and collaborative effort. We are especially grateful to our contributors for their forebearance in considering all our suggestions when revising their chapters, and for meeting deadlines so cheerfully. Any remaining errors or omissions are our own.

Sara Arber and Jay Ginn

1

'ONLY CONNECT': GENDER RELATIONS AND AGEING

Jay Ginn and Sara Arber

Gender and ageing are inextricably intertwined in social life; each can only be fully understood with reference to the other. As we age, we are influenced by the societal, cultural, economic and political context prevailing at different times in our life course. We are also profoundly influenced by our gender and by shifts in gender relations over the life course. Thus the connectedness of gender and ageing stems both from social change over time and from age-related life course events; social history and personal biography are interwoven over time. Yet ageing and gender have not been integrated in sociological thought and have rarely been researched in terms of their combined influence. At the macro level, we need to understand how age and gender are related to the distribution of power, privilege and well-being in society; and at the micro level, how age and gender contribute to identity, values, social networks and political and other affiliations.

This book aims to explore some of the linkages between ageing and gender by bringing together theorists and researchers who have considered both these dimensions of social life simultaneously. The title of this chapter 'Only Connect' (Forster 1989), signifies that in making connections between gender and ageing, the understanding of both can be enhanced. However, we recognize that connections need to be more wide-ranging, encompassing the interaction of gender and age with other bases of social differentiation, including class, race and ethnicity (Levy 1988).

In this chapter, we first examine the separation of gender and ageing in sociological theory and research, suggesting that there are parallels between the past neglect of gender and the current invisibility of ageing and later life in

British sociology. Next we consider how the insights of feminist work might help in the development of a sociological theory of ageing and gender. Finally, three meanings of age are distinguished, each of which have implications for gender relations. The term 'gender relations', by analogy with class relations, refers to the different position of men and women in the social hierarchy of power and status. In the course of the discussion we show how each of the book's chapters contributes to connecting gender and ageing.

The separation of gender and ageing

Although studies on older people usually take gender, as a variable, into account, the intersection of age relations and gender relations is under-developed in mainstream social theory (Levy 1988; Reinharz 1989; Arber and Ginn 1991b). Due to feminist influence it has been recognized that gender and class 'interact to form a new status that has elements of both but which is not reducible to either' (Morgan, D. 1986: 46); we argue that this also applies to gender and age relations. However, sociologists concerned with ageing and ageism have tended to 'add on' gender, treating it as a variable rather than integrating it as a fundamental relationship of social organization. At the same time, the predominant theoretical interest of academic feminists has until recently been concerned with how gender divisions in both the domestic sphere and the labour market contribute to the oppression of working age women, tending to neglect ageing and later life. This failure to connect gender and age theoretically seems odd in view of the fact that most older people are women, but may reflect the origin of second wave feminism, which began in a movement of mainly young women, a generational revolt. The lack of sociological research on older women is striking, given the richness of work by feminist sociologists, although recent research is beginning to redress this neglect (see Peace 1986; McDaniel 1989; Arber and Ginn 1991a; Bernard and Meade 1993). Like diners at separate tables, ageing theorists and feminist sociologists have been exchanging some meaningful glances but without pooling their conceptual resources.

In terms of methods, too, feminist sociology and social theory on ageing have used different approaches (McDaniel 1989); the former has been mainly theory-driven and qualitative, contextualizing women's experiences and concerned with achieving social change to improve women's visibility and social status. Research on ageing, in contrast, has tended to be quantitative, policy-driven and ameliorative (concerned with how individuals can adjust to their reduced social and physical status).

Over the last 20 years, feminist work has sought to transform male-dominated mainstream (or 'malestream') theory. Feminist sociologists showed that malestream sociology was not only sexist in omitting consideration of women in topics such as class mobility and class identity, but also that its conceptual and methodological tools were inappropriate for an adequate treatment of gender (Roberts 1981). A radical reorientation was required, in which gender was treated as a fundamental basis of stratification and in which issues that are central to the lives of women were integrated into theory. Just as feminist sociologists had to reconceptualize whole areas of sociology (Abbott and Wallace 1990), reconstructing existing sociological understanding is needed so that age relations as well as gender relations are integrated.

The methodological stance of feminism was crucial, especially in the early days (Roberts 1981; McRobbie 1982; Stanley and Wise 1983). The dominant approach was qualitative, to give an audience to previously unheard voices and to make visible what was previously unseen. The overriding concern was to take the perspective of women within the context of everyday life. An associated aim in early feminist methodology was to break down the barriers between the researcher and the researched, to reduce the power imbalance, and where possible to use the research to empower women (Oakley 1982; Reinharz 1983). These methodological imperatives have, however, inadvertently objectified older women as a burden to be cared for by working age women (Finch and Groves 1982; Nissel and Bonnerjea 1982; Lewis and Meredith 1988), as well as reinforcing the invisibility of older women and purveying negative images of ageing. Later quantitative research by feminists has begun to redress this by demonstrating the considerable contribution to caring for other older people made by older women and men (Arber and Ginn 1990). 'The personal is political' became a clarion call, associated with the recognition of how the researcher's own biography influenced the issues to be researched and the interpretation of research data, whether qualitative or quantitative. The methodological canons of feminist research need to be applied to research on later life, giving older women and men a voice, taking on their own perspectives as subjects rather than objects of research (Oakley 1981; Ribbens 1989).

The sociology of ageing lags well behind that of gender and has yet to become a recognized subfield within British sociology. It is still the case that 'the use of age in ways which are theoretically informed as well as empirically rigorous is relatively uncharted territory. Still less has age been developed as an important topic for research in its own right' (Finch 1986: 12). Although there is important sociological research on later life in Britain (for example Bytheway et al. 1989; Jefferys 1989), this work has been marginal to mainstream and feminist sociology. Extensive research in social policy relates to older people but this has tended to emphasize either the social problems of older people or, more negatively, older people as a social problem (Arber and Ginn 1991b). Insights from the sociology of ageing need to be integrated within mainstream sociology, and research on ageing needs to shift from a primarily social problem focus to encompass a broad range of sociological research issues.

The nascent state of the sociology of ageing can be judged from the lack of refinement of the term 'age'. In early feminist writing, a key distinction was made between sex, primarily reflecting biological differences, and gender, referring to the socially constructed nature of the gender roles and gender relations which structure society (Oakley 1982; Morgan, D. 1986). A distinction parallel to that between sex and gender needs to be made in relation to age, as we discuss later.

Developing a sociology of ageing and gender

Parallels can be seen between mainstream sociology's gender-blindness until the 1970s and the current invisibility of later life in sociology. Both stem from classical sociology's preoccupation with waged work, class formation and class conflict, at the expense of life outside the confines of the formal economy (Kohli 1988; Arber and Ginn 1991b). The ageing of societies is stimulating increasing interest in later life, but the danger is that age, like gender, will be subject to the 'add and stir' approach (Anderson 1983), in which age and gender are merely treated as separate and additive variables in analysis. Such an approach, because it tends to be insensitive to interactive processes and to ignore bias in the production of knowledge, is likely to oversimplify. Feminist sociologists early pointed out that attempting to redress the masculine bias of sociology by merely adding data about women was inadequate. Their work has transformed sociology since the early 1970s, with the result that gender now forms an integral part of mainstream sociology.

Feminist arguments about the necessity of reconceptualizing rather than 'adding on' gender to existing theory are extended to age by McMullin (Chapter 3). She argues that theoretical construction reflects power imbalances in society: those who are least powerful in economic terms, such as older women who are black or disabled, attract the least theoretical attention. If age and gender are to be fully integrated into sociological theory, they must be treated as fundamental to social organization. McMullin suggests ways in which this might be achieved by building a more comprehensive theory of social stratification derived from Acker's (1988) theoretical model. Since age, like gender, influences the means by which resources are distributed to the individual (from parents, through participation in production, from a partner or from the state), Acker's theory could usefully be extended to include age. Such a distributional framework was implicitly adopted in our analysis of how the material, health and caring resources of older people are structured according to gender, age, class and ethnicity, and how structured inequality in later life is related to women's earlier disadvantage in the labour market due mainly to the gender division of domestic labour (Arber and Ginn 1991a).

The question of how to construct a more explicit, coherent and sociological framework for gender and ageing is taken up by Bury (Chapter 2). Three main types of theory in the field of ageing are critically assessed for their neglect of gender. The structural (or political economy) approach is seen as over-emphasizing structural disadvantage (or dependency) at the expense of attention to older people's agency in resisting poverty and low status through social organization; macro level analysis tends to neglect cultural change as well as the diversity of cultural meanings among older people, and to render the voice of older people inaudible. In contrast, Laslett's (1989a) focus on the positive aspects of population ageing, encapsulated by the concept of the 'Third Age', highlights human agency, stressing the opportunities for personal growth and choice. However, as Bury points out, Laslett's vision is prescriptive rather than explanatory and is based on élitist assumptions. Bury's third theoretical strand, the life course perspective, has the advantage of a dynamic approach which recognizes the dual influences of social structure and cultural change, but, like Laslett's writing, life course approaches underplay social inequality in later life, including that between women and men. A sociological theory of ageing and gender, Bury concludes, needs to combine the dynamism and agency implicit in life course perspectives with a structural framework; this must include gender as a fundamental dimension of the social division, as well as class and ethnicity.

Three meanings of age

Most writing on ageing blurs the difference between several meanings of age, a lack of conceptual clarity which has hampered sociological understanding of ageing. In the same way that the distinction between sex and gender became a basic tenet of feminist research in the 1970s, we argue that an adequate sociological theory of age needs to distinguish between at least three different meanings – chronological age, social age and physiological age – and how they interrelate. Chronological (or calendar) age is essentially biological, but needs to be distinguished from physiological age, which is a medical construct, referring to the physical ageing of the body, manifest in levels of functional impairment. Social age refers to the social attitudes and behaviour seen as appropriate for a particular chronological age, which itself is cross-cut by gender. As Finch (1986: 24) comments, 'Clearly age is a social category with a biological basis, but biology tells us little about its social meaning and significance'. In all three meanings – chronological age, social age and physiological age – ageing is gendered (that is, it operates differently for women and men), and is also socially structured, as we illustrate below.

Chronological age

Chronological age refers to age in years. Ageing in this sense brings changes to one's structural position in society, due to the various responsibilities and privileges which depend on chronological age. Some of these are enshrined in law; for example, liability for military service, eligibility to vote and to claim state benefits all depend on age. Age-based institutions such as retirement exert constraints on behaviour, as emphasized by structured dependency theory (Walker 1980; Townsend 1981). However, age-based structural constraints may differ for women and men, for example in military obligations, in the age of homosexual consent, in the age of entitlement to vote (in the past) and in state pension age.

The sociology of ageing has been mainly concerned with later life, often defined by a chronological age of 65 and above. Sociological and social policy interest has centred on the consequences for society of population ageing, which has arisen from both declining fertility and increased longevity (Laslett 1987; Ermisch, 1990). 'Apocalyptic demography' (Clark 1993) has led to fears about rising costs of pensions and of health and welfare services used by older people, together with projections of a rising dependency ratio which has fuelled the portrayal of older people as a burden on taxpayers. The prevalence of these societal attitudes can be seen as a moral panic, often expressed in terms of 'intergenerational conflict', where older people, especially in the US, are blamed for the poverty of the young (Johnson *et al.* 1989). Such negative portrayals of older people reflect not only ageism but, since the majority of older people are women, sexism as well. Defining a social group as 'dependent' purely on the basis of chronological age ignores the wide diversity among older people, in terms of their employment status, material resources, their physiological age, their health, their lifestyles and social networks; it discounts older people's past contributions to the economy in working and paying taxes and the consequent legitimacy of their claim on later generations; and it also overlooks their unpaid contributions to society both in earlier life (Greene 1989) and in later life, in terms of grandparenting and volunteering, as well as informal care provided by older people, mainly to their spouse and neighbours (Arber and Ginn 1990). Older people's contribution through unpaid work to their own generation and to the younger generation is as invisible today as was the case 20 years ago for women's unpaid domestic and caring work.

Age of eligibility for state pensions interacts with the age difference between marital partners in influencing couples' retirement status. On average men marry women who are two years younger than themselves, and there is a cultural norm against men marrying older women. Patriarchal ideology supports the dominance of husbands over wives, which is expressed in gender differences in the age of husbands and wives, and the norm of financial dominance of husbands over wives (Arber and Ginn 1995a). If state policy on pensionable age were to encourage women and men to retire at the same age, wives would be employed, on average, for two years after their husbands had retired, threatening male financial dominance. Thus gender inequality in state pension age, institutionalized in many European Union (EU) countries, may be seen as a response to the interaction of gender and age in marital relationships. The way in which British couples' retirement timing, in the context of unequal state pension ages, depends on their age difference, their health and other factors is the subject of Chapter 6 by Arber and Ginn. The difference in men's and women's state pension age in Britain tends to facilitate the traditional pattern of retirement timing by compensating for the marriage age differential.

Social age

The meaning of social age is in some ways comparable to the concept of gender; it is socially constructed and refers to age norms as to appropriate attitudes and behaviour, subjective perceptions (how old one feels) and ascribed age (one's age as attributed by others). Age-based norms, like gender norms, are maintained by ideologies which are resistant to change. For example, the notion that abilities, especially learning capacity, decline with age is deeply entrenched, in spite of a lack of evidence to support the belief (Clennell 1987). Such a prejudice serves to legitimate the social institution of retirement based on chronological age.

Social ageing is related to transitions in the life course, but since the timing and sequencing of such transitions differs for women and men (and according to class and ethnicity), social ageing is gendered. Because of cultural norms about reproductive roles women's working lives follow a different pattern from men's – a 'female chronology' (Itzin 1990a). In terms of desirability as partners, women are often said to be 'over the hill' or 'past their sell-by date' at an earlier age than men; attitudes to women as partners become more negative, whereas ageing in men is more acceptable – a double standard of ageing (Sontag 1978). A similar process occurs in the labour market, where women's opportunities are jeopardized by employers' and managers' prejudices. As one writer in the US summed up research evidence, 'Older women face the same problem as older workers in general, but to a greater extent and earlier in the life course' (Rodeheaver 1990: 104).

Most research on age–gender discrimination in employment has been North American (for example, Leonard 1982; McConnell 1983; Hess 1986; Herz and Rones 1989). Bernard *et al.* (Chapter 5) use British data to examine the ways in which such gendered ageism operates to women's disadvantage in their employment and retirement. The position of older staff in local government was studied through a national survey, while the views of a small sample of older women in public and private organizations were also elicited. Bernard *et al.* show how age and gender in combination disadvantage women in the labour market; how a 'glass ceiling' limiting women's careers arises from managers' attitudes to women's ageing; how women may internalize low expectations as to their own capabilities in mid-life; and how gendered processes in the labour market also diminish women's chances of accumulating an adequate pension. An important effect of the lesser desirability of older women as employees is that the gap between men's and women's earnings widens with age (Taueber and Valdisera 1986). Since most occupational pensions depend on final salary (as well as on years of pensionable service), this contributes to women's lower income in later life (Ginn and Arber 1994b). The shorter employment records and lower average pay of women means that the pension consequences of mid-life divorce are more serious for women than for men (Ginn and Arber 1991). Thus social age, as well as chronological age, contributes to structural disadvantage, but in different ways for women and men.

Some have argued that in postmodern society social age is becoming more fluid; norms as to the timing of work and education have become more flexible (Hirschorn 1977) or should do (Laslett 1987, 1989a; Handy 1991), while dress and leisure activities are less closely tied to chronological age than in the past (Featherstone and Hepworth 1989). According to this view, normative expectations about appropriate lifestyles among older people are weakening as improved health enables more people to have a Third Age of active leisure between retirement and the onset of frailty (Laslett 1987). It is important to remember, however, that the rosy scenario of a Third Age of self-development, autonomy, consumption and youthful lifestyles is essentially a bourgeois option, unavailable to those who have low incomes or poor health. As Bury points out (Chapter 2), Laslett's approach tends to neglect structural inequality and the way material and cultural factors influence the meaning and actual experience of life transitions. Age-based norms may still exert powerful pressure to 'act one's age', especially among less advantaged social groups.

The Third Age appears to offer opportunities for older women to develop other identities than that of wife, mother or paid worker, through engaging in leisure, social and other activities. In practice, however, older women continue to be more occupied than men with domestic and family obligations, especially if they are married, so that they have less 'free time' than retired men (see Chapter 5 and Bernard and Meade 1993). As for men, class and ethnicity influence older women's opportunity and desire to redirect their energies at this stage of life but for some women, socialization into gender roles, often barely questioned in young adulthood, may be challenged and resisted as they age (McDaniel 1988). As one group of older women have declared, they are now free to 'grow old disgracefully';

> the conditions of our lives have dictated that we repress our own dreams and desires in order to tend to everyone else's . . . when our web of family and work obligations is shrinking, we can seize the opportunity to actualize what we were only able to dream during years of self-denial.
>
> (Hen Co-op 1993: 106)

It is this possibility of finding an 'authentic' self as opposed to conforming to socially prescribed roles which is explored by Ingrisch (Chapter 4). She examines the life histories of three middle class older Austrian women in order to understand how they perceived and dealt with conflicts between their own aspirations and the behaviour expected of them. Their differing responses were influenced both by shifts in the ideological climate over time and by their own experience of work and family over the life course, yet in later life each had reached some resolution of earlier conflicts.

The life histories analysed by Ingrisch remind us that social ageing does not occur in a static environment; in particular, the socially prescribed female chronology varies over time and place. The historical period of early socialization has been said to exert a disproportionately powerful influence over attitudes and expectations (Mannheim 1952); gender relations in different cohorts tend, therefore, to differ according to the gender ideology, military demands, economic climate and so forth prevailing in their youth, mediated additionally by class relations and ethnicity. If social change is minimal, gender norms are likely to be reinforced in adulthood by the peer group and by the older generation. However, rapid social change may modify norms established in young adulthood. The far-reaching changes this century in reproductive technology (especially the contraceptive pill), the expansion of women's opportunities in education and employment, changed attitudes to marital relationships and parenthood, the social movements concerned with race and gender equality and citizenship rights for disadvantaged social groups, the shifting needs of capitalism for men's and women's labour and the backlash against feminism and collectivism have been experienced by different cohorts at varying stages in their life course. How far men and women move with the times as they age, adapting their gender relationships in response to such changes, or adhere to attitudes and behavioural patterns established earlier is not clear.

The life course as it evolves invites change in gender roles and relationships, as the material basis of the gender division of labour in employment and childrearing changes. In later life, when these roles have been largely lost, older people could be said to inhabit not only a Third Age but also (in spite of being active members of society and important as consumers), a 'third sphere' (Carlsen and Larsen 1993), which is neither production nor reproduction. The question of whether later life brings greater equality of roles between husbands and wives, and if so, whether this shifts power in marital relationships towards women, is an intriguing one. Some writers have suggested this is so (for example, Friedman 1987), but it may depend on whether married women have been able to acquire independent pension income. Although the breadwinner role, in terms of wage-earning, ends with retirement, husbands' pension income in most countries is much higher than women's (Ginn and Arber 1991, 1992, 1994a, 1994b), which would contribute to perpetuating men's relative power in marriage into later life.

Research on how gender roles, attitudes and expectations develop with ageing suggests gender convergence, or a tendency towards androgyny (Rossi 1986; Sinnott 1986); gender roles become less sharply defined in the latter half of life, with older men showing more affiliative, nurturant tendencies than younger, while older women are more independent and assertive than younger (Rossi 1980; Gutmann 1987). The traditional domestic division of labour into 'feminine' (especially laundry, cleaning, cooking) and 'masculine' tasks (mainly repairs and maintenance of home, garden and car, where these exist) is reported by some researchers in the US to diminish with age (for example, Sinnott 1977). However, research on middle-class couples in mid-life and later life demonstrated that household tasks were still strongly sex-linked; retired men and women both had greater involvement in masculine tasks than employed people and men participated more in feminine tasks after retirement. Interestingly, taking on cross-sex tasks was linked with greater well-being for women but not for men (Keith and Schafer 1982), consistent with Oakley's (1974) contention that housework is unsatisfying. Although Gutmann attributed gender convergence to hormonal changes, the chapters in this book show that women themselves explain their new-found energy and outgoingness in later life as springing from the diminution of obligatory family roles.

Research on marital roles in later life is reviewed by Askham (Chapter 7); she argues that more sophisticated models of marriage are needed, in which power and authority are adequately theorized. In addition, when assessing processes in long term marriages it is important to distinguish the effects of ageing and long association of the couple from cohort effects, recognizing the very different historical circumstances in which older and younger people had their most influential socializing experiences.

The way that married couples in advanced old age had modified their gender roles, and how these differed from those of single and previously married older people is explored by Wilson through in-depth interviews with a sample of Londoners aged over 75 (Chapter 8). This research showed that gender roles between spouses had become blurred, with men conforming less closely to a masculine stereotype in terms of tasks performed; however, some gender inequality of power persisted in the marital relationship. Widowers were more likely to look forward to remarriage than widows, the latter seeing advantages in having friendships with men but preferring to remain free of women's traditional servicing role in marriage. Thus although widowhood for women is usually associated with a drop in household income, widows gain the freedom to budget as they choose, and despite losing a lifelong companion, some women may welcome the release from tiresome routine work.

Physiological age

A third meaning of age refers to the physiological ageing process. Although related to chronological age, the medical construct of physiological age cannot be simply read off from age in years. Physiological age relates to functional ability and the gradual decline in bone density, muscle tone and strength which occurs with advancing age. However, the speed and timing of these physiological changes varies according to position in the social structure, especially gender and class (Arber and Ginn 1991a; 1993b). Both Laslett's (1989a) discussion of the Fourth Age as characterized by 'dependence, decrepitude and death' and use of the concept of 'deep old age' by cultural theorists such as Featherstone and Hepworth (1989) are marking off these categories of older people based on physiological decline. Blaikie argues that the Fourth Age is increasingly becoming separated from the Third Age and is stigmatized, the subject of fear and taboo. He suggests that 'perhaps deep old age will become the great prohibition of the twenty-first [century]?' (1994: 6–7).

Gender differences in mortality, as well as in the prevalence, type and age of onset of disabilities are all associated with physiological ageing, and give rise to significant gender imbalances in later life. Because women outlive men by an average of six years, there are 50 per cent more women than men among those aged over 65. The gender imbalance is most marked in advanced old age; over age 85, women outnumber men by three to one. The fact that half of older women are widowed, whereas three-quarters of older men are married, has consequences for gender identity, relationships and roles in later life (Arber and Ginn 1991a).

Poor health or disability have implications for relationships between spouses and between parents and their adult children, because of the loss of independence of the person being cared for and the stress that attention to their needs imposes on the carer. Because of gender differences in disability and the numerical imbalance of women and men in later life, the provision and receipt of informal care are gendered. Older women are more likely than older men to have their activities of daily living impaired by functional disabilities, yet women are far less likely to have a spouse to provide care and enable them to remain living in the community (Arber and Ginn 1991a). Whereas men can largely rely on their wives when care is required, with all the advantages this brings, women more often have to call upon adult children for help and are twice as likely as men to enter residential care. Little is understood about how physical and mental frailty affect the gendering of power in marital and other kin relationships.

The way older spouses deal with a shifting balance of need and care between them is the subject of the chapter by Rose and Bruce (Chapter 9). From a postal survey of 2,000 older people in a multicultural city in the North of England, they focus on the experience of 16 couples where one of the partners was substantially disabled. The method of interviewing – simultaneous but separate – ensured that each partner was able to give an autonomous view of the caring relationship. Men, whether carers or cared-for, tended to stay in control. As carers, men were willing to set aside gender norms as to appropriate tasks in order to preserve the independence of the couple, but in doing so they saw themselves as 'Mr. Wonderful', admired for their competence by all concerned. In contrast, older women, who performed equally heroic tasks to maintain the ideology of the independent and mutually supportive couple, saw what they did as obligatory; this view was shared by those around them, thus giving little social esteem to the care work of older women.

Frailty associated with physiological ageing affects not only marital relationships but also wider social support networks; the way different types of network shift in response to increasing disability and need for assistance is shown by Scott and Wenger (Chapter 12). The impact of increasing frailty on support networks was not the same for women and men, the former depending more on their adult children and the latter, due to earlier mortality, relying mostly on their wives.

Martin Matthews and Campbell (Chapter 10) consider the gender implications of care provision by adult children, analysing the effects on employment of women and men who care for elderly relatives in Canada. Data on eldercare responsibilities and career opportunity costs was collected from over 5,000 employees. They show that women were much more likely than men to provide informal care and in addition that the adverse effects on career opportunities of providing care were greater for women employees than for men. Gender differences in career costs were, however, less pronounced among those providing more intensive, personal care.

The context in which care is mainly provided, whether from relatives living elsewhere, within the household, from social services or within an institution, will affect the extent of an older person's independence and power; who provides care, in terms of the nature of the kin relationship, may also be relevant. Loss of autonomy is more obvious for those living in a residential institution, where staff have control over most aspects of their existence, than for older people living at home. In either context, however, tension and conflict between carers and cared-for may develop into elder abuse, in terms of verbal cruelty, neglect or violence. Older women's greater likelihood of being widowed means that they are more dependent than older men on adult children for care and also more likely to live in an institution; these different contexts may give rise to gender differences in the incidence of abuse. Although feminist researchers have clarified our understanding of family conflict and violence at earlier stages of the life course, they have not turned their attention to elder abuse. Whittaker (Chapter 11) discusses the emphasis on definitional and measurement problems in her review of research and theory on elder abuse. She argues that a tendency by writers to define and theorize elder abuse in terms of family dysfunction has obscured the gendered power relationships which are involved in elder abuse, especially the greater propensity of men to use violence, whether as carers or cared-for. Abuse must be located in an analysis of power relationships and gender is central to this analysis (Wilson 1994).

A number of issues relevant to gender and social ageing remain unexplored in this book. For example, little is known about how the experience of ethnic minorities or of gays and lesbians may differ from that of the majority population. Although the negative stereotyping of older women includes lesbians (MacDonald and Rich 1984), they may be better able than other women to avoid the adverse effects (Berger 1982), having resisted conventional gender socialization which places a high value on youthfulness and femininity in women. Gender differences cross-cut sexual orientation. It is likely that among working age women, disadvantages in the labour market apply equally to lesbians, with similar adverse effects on their income in later life. Older lesbians may retain a wider support network of friends than gays, because of the latter's greater likelihood of engaging in shorter-term relationships. Among ethnic minority elders, ageing in a second homeland without the support of an extended family may be experienced as more isolating for women than for men, especially where language barriers exist (Bhalla and Blakemore 1981). These issues need further attention to balance the predominant focus in ageing research on heterosexual white women and men.

Conclusion: Integrating gender and age

Western societies are ageing and later life is dominated by women, yet gender and age relations have been traditionally ignored by mainstream sociological theory, both separately and in terms of their intersection. Feminist scholars rarely consider age relations, and theorists of ageing tend to 'add on' gender without rethinking assumptions and categorizations based on men as the reference group. This separation of gender and age in sociology hampers understanding of the many ways in which the process and social significance of ageing has different implications for women and men.

Gender relations cannot be assumed to be static over the life course, since life transitions, age-based norms and physiological changes all impact on the way gender roles are constructed and gender identity experienced.

If we are to understand ageing in society, it is important first to develop a sociological theory which can adequately encompass both gender and age, distinguishing the several meanings of age – chronological age, social age and physiological age. Of course, an adequate theoretical framework must allow for other significant sources of differentiation besides age and gender, such as class, ethnicity and historical time of birth, all of which contribute to the accumulating diversity among older people.

Research methods need to capture the rich diversity of ageing and provide a sociological understanding building on the perspectives of older women and men. It is vital that quantitative research *on* older people is balanced by research *with* older people, in which older people are the subjects of research and their perspectives and concerns orient the research. In this book, a range of research methods is represented, with many of the chapters based on qualitative work in which older people are studied as active subjects and given a voice.

In the following chapters, ways to achieve a better theorization of age and gender are suggested; assessments of existing conceptualization and knowledge about gender roles, power and ageing are provided; and new research in this area is presented. We show that gender roles and identities which have developed in earlier phases of the life course through patriarchal practices in the family, labour market and state, continue to structure women's and men's relationships in later life. However, some of these patriarchal structures become less prominent, particularly those associated with reproduction and the labour market, while others are becoming increasingly evident, particularly the gendered nature of state policies in later life (to which we return in the final chapter). Thus there are cross-cutting influences on older women's and men's lives, some tending to reduce women's oppression, some serving to maintain it as in earlier phases of the life course and others to increase it.

Age and gender are intimately linked in social life and our aim has been to begin to reconnect them in sociological thinking and research. A great deal more research is needed to explain how the place of older women in society is related to both patriarchy and capitalism. We hope that this book will stimulate further contributions, in terms of theory and research, to the task of reconnecting age and gender.

2

AGEING, GENDER AND SOCIOLOGICAL THEORY

Mike Bury

The last 15 years have witnessed an unprecedented rise in interest and debate about ageing, despite the frequent charge that the subject has been neglected in academic as well as public life. Indeed, it has sometimes seemed that hardly a day has gone by during this period without another book being published, or another course or journal being launched. Writing and research on social aspects of ageing, or social gerontology, continues to expand, including calls for more critical perspectives to incorporate such issues as class, gender and ethnicity.

Despite this expansion it is also frequently alleged that much of the work in the ageing field has been policy oriented, and, indeed policy driven, as governments and non-governmental agencies have attempted to address the never ending 'problems' that an ageing population appears to create. As a result, the field of ageing has remained theoretically underdeveloped; as an apparently 'applied' field of study theory has remained in the back seat. Fennell *et al.* comment, for example, that theoretical developments in social aspects of ageing have at best had a 'chequered history' (1988: 41). It might also be argued that more recent programmatic statements calling for 'new perspectives' to meet this criticism run the risk of becoming what Dressel (1991) refers to as a 'mix and stir approach' where the latest information on various dimensions of experience (and especially disadvantage) in old age are simply added to the standard recipe. Evidence on gender and ethnicity, for example, may appear as afterthoughts creating a long-running litany of woe, without being integrated fully into a developing framework.

Though this may well be an important criticism of some of the recent contributions in social gerontology, this chapter will try to show that new and more coherent approaches to ageing *have* begun to develop in recent years, but they have paid insufficient attention to its gendered character. However, in order to evaluate these developments in the light of the criticisms mentioned above, there is a need to adopt a more explicit theoretical framework. The adoption of such a framework may help not only in mapping recent developments, but also suggest ways in which linkages between different aspects of ageing might be strengthened.

The argument here is that the call for a more theoretically consistent approach to age and ageing should be more specific about what kind of theory is needed. Even writers such as Fennell *et al.* while making their point about the chequered history of theory in ageing, seem rather unclear what they actually mean by this. At one point, for example, they talk of 'social theory' and then two pages later 'social gerontological theory' (Fennell *et al.* 1988: 41,42) without clarifying what kind of *conceptual framework* is being invoked.

Following Mouzelis (1991), I suggest that an adequate *sociological*, as opposed to a general 'social' approach needs to address the relationship between micro and macro levels of analysis, the nature of the links between agency and structure, and especially focus on the notion of *social hierarchies*. From this viewpoint, class, gender and ethnicity, as features of hierarchical social relations at a macro level (for example, in their influence over policy formation and implementation by the state), and as part of micro interactions at a local or community level, would come into sharper focus. Mouzelis (1991) makes the point that 'social interaction' is often wrongly conflated with micro level analysis alone, whereas the main point concerns the *consequences* of inter-action, with macro level interactions (e.g. among government ministers over setting benefit or pension levels) having a wider impact than those at a micro level.

The examination of the relationship between agency and structure is important in developing a perspective on ageing, since it challenges the portrayal of older people (especially women) as passive victims of circum-stance. This chapter argues that gender and ageing can be theorized more adequately if approached in this way, and as a key part of the sociological enterprise. Without the employment of an explicit conceptual framework, calls for a more 'critical' social gerontology are likely to remain unanswered.

The chapter reviews three main areas of work on the sociology of ageing, particularly with respect to their implications for an understanding of its 'gendered' character. These are: structural or 'political economy' approaches to ageing and dependency; Laslett's theory of the Third Age; and approaches focusing on biography and the life course. The main lines of argument developed in each of these sections is outlined, followed by comments on their adequacy at the level of sociological theory. Finally, the threads are drawn together by arguing for a more explicit and general approach to the sociology of gender and ageing.

Structured dependency in ageing

Throughout the 1960s and 70s a series of reactions to the prevailing functionalist analysis of a range of social problems occurred. Ageing was no exception. The dominance of a functionalist view of ageing as a form of social disengagement and, in terms of role theory, as the progressive loss of roles (Havinghurst 1954; Cumming and Henry 1966) became the focus of a sustained challenge from sociologists and policy analysts, both in the United States and in the UK.

Two main objections were made to the functionalist position. First, it was seen to act as a convenient ideological weapon, justifying arguments about the increasingly 'problematic' status of an ageing population, and the need to take action to limit the putative 'burden' that the non-productive 'disengaged' elderly created, especially calls on the public purse. Second, and concomitantly, it stressed the importance of personal adjustment by the individual. The loss of roles involved through retirement from an active working life (activism being one of the most dominant 'functional' social values — particularly linked to the position of the working man) and the physical and mental deterioration associated with advancing age (particularly among women) ran the risk, it was argued, of a progressive 'ego centredness', or self-absorbtion, developing in old age.

Though there have been recent arguments for retaining at least some aspects of the disengagement perspective (Fennell *et al.* 1988), especially with respect to the 'oldest old' (Johnson and Barer 1992), a series of counter-arguments were put forward in the 1970s and 1980s which sought to relocate the problems of dependency and ageing in social structural, rather than individual, terms. For the sake of brevity the discussion here focuses on just two examples from the early 1980s by Townsend (1981) and Walker (1981), and subsequent arguments by Estes (1986) and Walker (1987) which brought gender more fully into the picture.

In contrast to functionalist views of the low social status and 'adjustment' problems of the elderly, Townsend (1981) counterposed a perspective in which he emphasized the social creation, or manufacture of dependency. The term 'structured dependency', derived from this, attempted to shift attention away from the characteristics of individuals to those of the wider social system. In particular, to use Mouzelis' (1991) terms, Townsend focused on the 'rules and resources' governing ageing in modern capitalist societies and the main ways in which they express themselves.

Townsend drew attention to four main sources of 'structured dependency': the effects of retirement policies, especially on late middle-aged workers in a period of high unemployment; the presence of widespread poverty in which nearly half of the elderly are portrayed as 'in poverty' or 'on the margins'; the negative effects of residential care; and the tendency of community care policies to create what Townsend called 'grateful and passive recipients' (1981: 22). He then marshalled a variety of empirical evidence in support of these contentions. In his conclusion Townsend pointed to the 'structure and organisation of production' as the source of these dependency features. Arguing against the 'pluralist tradition' of writing on ageing, he called for a 'political economy' approach which would combine 'sociological, economic and political analyses'.

Walker (1981, 1987) in the UK, and Estes (1986, 1991) in the US, took up a similar theme, arguing for a 'political economy of old age'. Their main point was that in order to understand the position of elderly people in modern capitalist societies, the main determining factor on quality of later life is the influence of adult labour market position through and after retirement.

Walker argued that earlier writers had treated age and ageing with an implicit assumption that the elderly were a 'distinct social group'. 'Rather than concentrating on the biologically based differences in ageing and individual adjustments to the ageing process' (1987: 179) Walker called for attention to the 'social creation' of dependency, the structural relationship between different age groups and the impact of the division of labour and the labour market on the elderly (Walker 1981: 77). Estes, in a similar vein, called for a political economy approach to ageing as being 'conditioned by one's location in the social structure and the relations generated by the economic mode of production and the gendered nature of the division of labor' (Estes 1991: 21). This led to an examination of the impact of retirement and disablement on older people, and their links with poverty and inequality in later life. The main conclusion of these analysts was that the effects of a weak position in the labour market, prior to retirement, meant restricted access to 'a wide range of resources' and resulted in 'the imposition of depressed social status' (Walker 1981: 88) in old age. Estes concluded that 'the future of ageing in the US will be profoundly shaped by the economic, social and political crisis of capitalism' (Estes 1986: 132).

There is little doubt that the arguments and analysis put forward by Townsend, Walker and Estes drew attention to a set of important issues, which have had a significant impact on academic and public debate. Macnicol (1990), for example, has provided a useful summary of the subsequent challenges to the structured dependency argument, primarily from a social policy perspective. However, it is with the *sociological* character of the structured dependency argument, and its inadequate treatment of women, that the present discussion is concerned.

As stated, the 'structured dependency' position highlights important macro issues, especially, the rules and resources that influence and constrain everyday life for elderly people. In Estes's work, the role of the state in these processes receives particular attention. As a result, age and ageing emerge as important features of contemporary society, and not just as a field of study to which social analysis can be applied. As a corrective to the individualism of earlier approaches to ageing, and as a means of bringing the political dimension back in, the approach works well. However, it displays certain limits when approached from a more explicitly sociological viewpoint.

First, the emphasis on structural factors tends to be at the expense of any linkages with more micro processes, though it should be noted that Estes (1991) does attempt to bridge the gap. Mostly, however, retirement, poverty and pensions are discussed with little reference to the actual views people in different social groups hold about such matters, or how they may have changed over time. Having criticized the view of the elderly as 'homogeneous', it then creeps back in, in the sense that the voices of elderly people are rarely heard in these analyses, or used as a check on the assertions made. Nor are collective actions to influence policies in these areas analysed in any detail. Indeed, Townsend falls back on a rather ill-defined notion of agency when he says that public perceptions of the elderly and dependency are 'tempered by the restorative mechanism of the family' (1981: 13) without addressing the theoretical weakness of assuming the presence of traditional family structures. Though social action at a 'local' level is implied in such arguments, the question of agency is poorly specified compared with the detailed examination of policy issues. In particular, women, both as older people and as carers, appear as passive victims of circumstance. Walker's paper (1987) contains a catalogue of problems adding up to the view that 'elderly people and women in particular . . . are in effect trapped in poverty' (Walker 1987: 191), unsustained by any critical analysis.

The result of the overemphasis on structural factors produces a form of functionalism of its own. As Mouzelis points out, 'institutional analysis always implies functionalist analysis' (1991: 62) if the logical relationship between different structural elements within a system are to be understood. From this viewpoint the emphasis on labour market position in Walker and Estes underscores important common features of retirement, income and pensions, and therefore inequalities in old age. But the institutional linkages are only specified in the following generalized ways: 'poverty in old age is primarily a function of low economic and social status prior to retirement' and 'early retirement is primarily a function of socio-economic status' (Walker 1981: 74, 85). The attempt to overcome a functionalist analysis fails because of a reliance on a formalistic approach to social structure and its impact.

In order to produce a more sociologically consistent view of these relationships, an explicit use of the concept of *social hierarchies* is needed. If this conceptual focus was adopted, the vertical features of structures and the links between different levels of action – e.g. between policy makers, politicians, organizations and pressure groups of the elderly, as well as between different groups of women and men – would come into clearer view. As a result, links between structure and agency, for example, the changing nature of struggles over retirement in different periods, and the meaning it has for different social groups, would receive greater attention than they do. Without such a framework the reader is left feeling that nothing much has changed, or is ever likely to do so. Indeed, social change is curiously absent from structured dependency arguments.

This theoretical problem also has implications for the treatment of gender in these analyses. Though writers such as Townsend and Walker mention the position of women in their work, this too, is undertheorized. While earlier discussions of retirement and role loss focused almost entirely on the male worker, with females relegated to a consideration of their domestic roles in old age, current debates of the political economy variety still tend to introduce data on gender differences only in a limited way.

The failure to recognize gender relationships as a central feature of social hierarchy and of patterns of domination particularly hampers the analysis of Walker and Townsend, though this is less marked in Estes. Differences in life circumstances between men and women may not be simply a function of the differential impact of the labour market, but part of a set of culture-bound gendered relationships. Walker's attempt to address the gendered nature of the economic and social experience in old age, for example, is conceptualized as 'a line along which' such influences occur (Walker 1987: 178) rather than an expression of the *hierarchical* nature of imbalances in power between men and women. As a result, the impact of differences in status and power between men and women as well as the long term effects of patterns of female subordination are underestimated. For example, the reported higher life satisfaction in very old men (Bury and Holme 1991) may be as much to do with the generally higher status of men throughout the life course, compared with women, and the fact that very old men are more likely to be married than women of a comparable age, matters that are only in part a function of occupational status or retirement itself. And, as Gans (1992) has pointed out, hierarchical relationships and inequalities *among* women may be missed out altogether, for 'while working class women may have their differences with working class men, they also have differences with upper-middle class women' (Gans 1992: vii).

The adoption of a more conceptually adequate approach to structured dependency would have another benefit, namely to counteract its tendency to reinforce negative views of ageing and gender. The constant reiteration of the links between older people and dependency, poverty, inequality and low status runs the risk of reinforcing negative perceptions (especially of poorer older women), even though the intention is clearly to raise their political profile. It is here that greater attention to the relationship between agency and structure, and to micro as well as macro levels of analysis, would offer a more consistent sociological way forward, by insisting that the documentation of problems be matched by evidence on how people tackle them. Without such an approach, human agency and the meaning of ageing tends to be left out of the analysis.

This approach is particularly important at a time of radical restructuring in the economic and social spheres, where the 'rules and resources' governing the elderly are changing rapidly, and where active responses are being fashioned by elderly people to meet them. For example, Williams's (1990) work on lay beliefs about health and dependency among older people stresses how 'dependency' is experienced in terms of moral imperatives, fashioned and drawn upon by different generations in different ways, as well as by economic factors. Jerrome's (1989) work on the active nature of friendship and social support in later life also demonstrates older people's active engagement in fashioning 'social circumstances' within varying moral and cultural contexts. The integration of such work into the structured dependency approach would not only produce a more sociologically adequate account, but also avoid the paradox of reinforcing precisely the negative images that it sets out to challenge.

The Theory of the Third Age

In this section and the next, alternative approaches will be discussed that make an explicit attempt to bring agency into the analysis of old age, or at least explore the cultural dimensions of ageing in a changing society. These approaches contrast sharply with 'structured dependency', in that they set out to emphasize change and opportunity rather than the 'problems' associated with ageing, though elements of the political economy approach remain relevant to some versions, and to their evaluation.

In a series of publications, culminating with the book *A Fresh Map of Life* the historical sociologist, Peter Laslett (1989a) has developed an argument which challenges both disengagement and dependency theories. His stated aim has been to construct a more positive image of ageing in contemporary societies, (Laslett 1987, 1989a, 1989b) which, as we shall see, has particular implications for older women. Laslett's argument focuses on the 'unintended consequences' of the demographic transition (the historic change towards low fertility rates and increasing life expectancy, which in combination lead to an ageing of the population). This is virtually complete in most advanced industrial societies, and is taking on an accelerated pace in many developing countries. This age transformation, for Laslett, is an example of unplanned social change, consequent on secular trends which throw into relief new social issues and challenges.

The extent of these changes in the age structure of modern populations, requires, according to Laslett, a fundamental rethinking of prevailing concepts of ageing, specifically conceptions of the 'Ages of Man' (*sic*). In the past, those reaching adulthood could only hope to live out their biblical span of three score years and ten, if they were that fortunate. Such was the comparative rarity of doing so, that planning for old age was hardly necessary. Today, especially for women, whose average life expectancy at birth, in the UK and comparable countries, is now nearly 80 years, this becomes an urgent necessity.

Laslett envisages four stages of ageing consistent with these changes, prized loose from the chronologically fixed categories of the past. He summarizes them as follows:

First comes an era of dependence, socialization, immaturity and education; second an age of independence, maturity and responsibility, of earning and saving; third an era of personal fulfilment; and fourth an era of final dependence, decrepitude and death.

(Laslett 1989a: 4)

Though these 'ages' are not strictly related to chronological age, it is clear that they coincide with certain age-related structures and institutions. Entering and exiting from the labour market, for example, mark the transitions from the first to the second stage, and from the second to the third stage respectively. However, this approach may be seen in contrast to the 'structured dependency' view discussed above, where the state pension age has been seen until recently to be critical to the transition into old age. Now most commentators recognize that exit from the labour market may well occur before the state pension age.

From Laslett's viewpoint, it is the Third Age which represents what he calls the 'real novelty', both in the sense of referring to the new demographic realities, and as a challenge to developing new ways of living. The Third Age is seen as the 'apogee' of life, a period of creative fulfilment, freed from the constraints of the Second Age, but not yet under the shadow of the Fourth.

Laslett's model of ageing is cast in demographic, structural and subjective terms. The demographic basis of the Third Age stems from changes in the pattern of survival and improvements in the expectation of life, as well as reductions in the retirement age. Although some individuals have always survived into what might now be seen as the Third Age, *populations* can only be seen to be enjoying, or facing, a Third Age when 'enough people live well into the Second Age, such that they can 'expect to be able to go onto the Third Age'. By this Laslett means that they will have more than a 50 per cent chance of doing so (Laslett 1989a: 78). The main point of the Third Age is to draw attention to the relationship between improved survival into later life and the expectation in early adult life of reaching it.

The argument at the subjective, individual, level is more an exhortation than a calculation. Laslett calls for new attitudes to take advantage of the Third Age, and this is where his gendered approach emerges more clearly. The attitudes being called for are cast in terms of creativity, personal growth and 'above all, choice'. There is an urgent need to develop new roles, he argues, especially for women, who are more likely than men to enter and live through the Third Age. Laslett goes on to develop his point about women and ageing when he states that 'wearing black, looking submissive and regretful, being thankful that no new thing is to be expected from them – these are not attitudes that a woman in the Third Age would now wish to adopt' (Laslett 1989a: 71).

Laslett's approach to women is thus strongly voluntaristic in tone. It is the need to be active and positive that is seen to be the determining factor in 'successful' ageing. Even at younger ages, when women are in their childbearing years, they should be thinking of the future. Laslett opines that: 'At the age of twenty five . . . it is prudent to think of yourself as you will be at the age of seventy' (1989a: 73). Older people, especially women, are told that it is 'their duty to work out a role model' (Laslett 1989a: 71) on which the different attitudes mentioned above can be based. Without such a conscious awareness of ageing Laslett is fearful that 'conventions and precedents' will not be set for those entering the Third Age in the future. Without them, people (especially women) will not be prepared for the challenges of old age.

Laslett's 'theory of the Third Age', finally leads to a call to create new institutions, especially in the fields of education and employment (see also Young and Schuller 1991). The administrative categories of conventional retirement, and the age-related structures governing education, according to Laslett, no longer meet the needs of contemporary populations. Reiterating his arguments for the University of the Third Age, Laslett hopes to challenge images of ageing which have dominated later life in the past, and to provide the necessary structures for the active individual.

Whilst there is little doubt that ideas surrounding the Third Age also have had a considerable impact on public debates about ageing, their theoretical status remains ambiguous. For example, although Laslett wishes to avoid chronological age as much as possible, it is clear that the Fourth Age of 'decline and decrepitude' concerns those 'requiring the largest amount of support' who are largely those aged 85 and over (Laslett 1989a: 41) and are women. It is in comparison with this negative Fourth Age that the active Third Age can be seen in such a positive light. By theorizing dependency in this way Laslett is in danger of displacing negative views of ageing from the 'young old' to the 'old old', and thus particularly onto very old women. At a time when the focus of medical and policy attention has turned to the question of the 'oldest old' (Suzman *et al.* 1992) this is unfortunate. Activism may not always be the only recipe for a good quality of life, and evidence suggests that a more 'passive' lifestyle may be compatible with a good quality of life at an advanced age (Bury and Holme 1991).

One of the main difficulties is that Laslett's 'theory' is strongly *normative* in character. It is as much advocating what *should* be social attitudes towards ageing as providing theoretical 'ground clearing' about actual trends and developments. The strong advocacy of the Third Age stops Laslett seeing some of the difficulties in drawing and operating his new boundaries, and his emphasis on the creative aspects of the Third Age too readily conveys a thinly disguised set of élitist middle-class values. It is a moot point what values are to count as 'creative' in the ageing process. One wonders, for example, what relevance the emphasis on 'earning and saving' in the Second Age has to the millions of unemployed men and women in Europe at the present time. Moreover, women are less likely to have the financial resources for the creative endeavours envisaged by Laslett, and the idea of fashioning new roles may be circumscribed by the requirement to continue to perform domestic and caring roles, for example for grandchildren.

Theoretically, Laslett's historical sociology operates at such a general level that structural features of specific social systems, especially the 'rules and resources' discussed in the previous section, that influence the pattern of ageing, take a back seat. Laslett's desire to strike a positive note about ageing, or, at least some aspects of it, means that a consideration of structured dependency issues or the influence of social hierarchies seems all but absent. Most notably, Laslett's comments on gender are couched in terms of 'attitudes', not in terms of actual social relations between men and women, or between gender and class, or how these might shape experiences in later life. In particular, the Third Age theory is tied to the idea of retirement from paid employment, which leaves out of the picture women who may never 'retire' from their domestic roles, and may not have been in paid employment during much of the Second Age. The idea that the 'traditional demeanour' of women needs changing, is, in any event, already rather out of date, as consumerism begins to impact on lifestyles among men and women in old age (discussed later). The whole idea of the 'Ages of Man', even in its new version, sounds, from this viewpoint, not only sexist but anachronistic.

Whilst Laslett's Third Age theory sets out to provide a new map of the life course, this latter concept remains largely unexamined in his thesis. As a result, little connection is made with other work which is developing such a perspective, and Laslett's theory of life stages remains detached from current sociological thinking about ageing. As will be stressed in the next section, the concept of the life course is actually fast becoming the predominant focus of sociological work on ageing.

The life course, ageing and late modern cultures

Different approaches within a life course perspective have developed rapidly in recent years, partly in reaction to some of the theoretical shortcomings outlined in the previous sections of this chapter. Their aim has been to provide a more adequate basis for conceptualizing both the meanings attached to age among various groups and the social positions of people at different stages of life. This, in turn, reveals age and ageing as key dimensions of late modern societies. A life course perspective emphasizes diversity in experience, rather than the inevitability of dependency on the one hand, and collective experiences rather than individualistic 'attitudes', on the other.

A sociology of age, drawing on the idea of the life course, has emerged with an emphasis on two interrelated aspects: '(1) aging over the life course as a social process and (2) age as a structural feature of changing societies and groups, as both people and roles are differentiated by age' (Riley et al. 1988: 243). The resulting perspective is aimed at contributing directly to mainstream sociology and providing, in turn, a more adequate sociological approach to research on ageing, especially from a feminist viewpoint (Arber and Ginn 1991a). My aim in this final section is to provide a brief summary of two different types of life course analysis and to assess them in sociological terms: what might be called a 'dynamic' and a 'postmodern' view of ageing respectively.

The life course and the dynamics of ageing

One of the main uses of the life course as an organizing concept has been to develop the analysis of the sources and consequences of dependency, disability and inequality in later life, and especially their gendered dimensions. Arber and Evandrou, for example, state that the life course approach 'provides a framework for analyzing the various influences which contribute to the life experiences of different groups of individuals at particular phases of their lives' (1993: 9). Hockey and James (1993) argue that 'the term life course, rather than life cycle' is now used in order to emphasize new social divisions in modern society. They go on to argue that 'rather than a predictable passage through fixed stages' there is now more variability in experience (p. 1).

However, despite the emphasis on diversity, Arber and Evandrou (1993) also make it plain that 'structural and cultural constraints' influence the various transitions involved across the life course. The experiences of different cohorts are emphasized in an attempt to bring historical as well as temporal elements into the picture. Moreover, the lasting impact of values and experiences of people born in different periods and cultures offsets an over-emphasis on individual diversity, as well as on structural features.

While various structural influences, particularly 'financial and material resources' are highlighted, these are seen to interact with powerful sources of meaning, including those deriving from social status, in shaping experiences in later life. In recognizing the importance of labour market position and its influence on old age, for example, Arber and Evandrou argue that the acquisition of material resources is influenced by such factors as the 'experience of caring responsibilities' at different stages of the life course (1993: 25). Work on gender and the life course builds on the earlier work of family sociologists, such as Hareven and Adams (1982), in which an awareness of the different biographies of women and men was already evident.

In developing such a line of argument, recent feminist writers implicitly, if not explicitly, challenge the assumptions of structured dependency and Third Age theories of ageing. A clearer focus on gender brings the culturally constructed nature of the meanings and values that surround old age into sharper relief. To take another example, Arber and Evandrou point out that widowhood has different meanings for women and men, not only because it is much more common among the former, but because a whole pattern of social relationships, including friendship, differ between the sexes. 'Age-appropriate' behaviour between women and men in widowhood has been constructed in very different ways (1993: 25) largely, until now, to the disadvantage of women.

An analysis of the cultural dimensions of ageing, in this way, helps to overcome a tendency towards a formalistic view of structure and dependency on the one hand, and an individualistic emphasis on 'attitudes' towards ageing, as in the Third Age theory, on the other. The promise of a more 'dynamic' approach aims to reconcile the influences of social structure and cultural change.

Postmodernism and the life course

The cultural dimensions of ageing are given particular attention in the second main approach to the life course, but from a different viewpoint. This approach examines how contemporary patterns of ageing reflect and contribute to a 'postmodern culture', rather than attempting to reconcile structural and meaning issues, as exemplified by Arber and Evandrou (1993). Thus this second approach aims to explore ageing as a critical dimension of cultural change.

In a series of papers and articles, Featherstone and Hepworth have outlined an approach which aims to 'de-construct', as much as construct a life course perspective on ageing (Featherstone and Hepworth 1989, 1991). Following writers such as Kohli (Kohli and Meyer 1986; Kohli 1988) who question the continuing centrality of the work ethic, and thus, by implication, the determining role of labour market position in the life course, particularly in the light of changing retirement patterns, Hepworth and Featherstone make a number of critical points.

Rejecting the idea of a fixed set of stages of the life course, these writers examine how the concept of the life course as a social institution arose. Following writers such as Giddens (1994: 5), who state that the development of modern society involves the reform of traditional patterns of behaviour and the emergence of clearer 'divisions between the sexes' with stability in certain 'normal' canons of sexual behaviour, it can be argued that age-relevance became more prominent than in the past. This also involves an extension of professional 'surveillance, control and normalisation' over the individual, emphasizing areas such as 'growth and development' (Featherstone and Hepworth 1989: 144) and the problems of 'middle age' and 'old age'. They argue, however, that 'postmodern change . . . will lead to some blurring' of these life stages. In this they echo, but go beyond, the Third Age theory and the life course approach discussed above, arguing that life stages are being radically reconstructed under the impact of demographic and social change.

Featherstone and Hepworth suggest a much more fluid picture than has been discussed so far. While writers, such as Townsend, reject the idea that the social structure is becoming increasingly 'pluralistic', and emphasize 'the inexorable process by which the status of older people has been lowered' (Townsend 1981: 6), Featherstone and Hepworth posit the emergence of what they call the 'de-hierarchicisation and pluralism' of postmodern cultures, bringing forward the possibility that chronological age will continue 'to be discredited as an indicator of inevitable age norms and life styles', with significant new values taking their place. Among these Featherstone and Hepworth highlight three main features.

First, they emphasize the 'cultivation of lifestyles' and consumerism among a wide range of age groups. Age need not be a barrier, for example, to health promotion activities, even though it once may have been (Bury *et al.* 1994). People, will, according to Featherstone and Hepworth, 'continue to deny the need to slow down, to rest, to take a back seat' (1991: 374). Second, a 'youthful approach to culture' is emerging in which the media and tourism offer pleasurable 'simulations' which cut across earlier age barriers, and where people in later life can enjoy pleasures not thought appropriate to older people in the past – the development of a kind of 'last of the summer wine' scenario (Martin 1990).

Third, new social movements will emerge, in which 'post-scarcity values' will be articulated, reflecting these new interests and preoccupations among older people. Women, in particular, will advance their interests, participating as 'valid partners' on the social scene (Featherstone and Hepworth 1989: 145–6). This, arguably, marks a shift towards the 'feminization of culture' as matters such as health, sexuality and domestic life (including negative aspects such as abuse and violence in families) emerge from the private into the public sphere and thus provide the basis for advancing the position of women (Featherstone 1992). The needs and activities of older women can be included here, as the developing 'discourse' on 'elder abuse' testifies (see Whittaker's Chapter 11). It should be noted at this point that gender has not been a central aspect of most postmodernist writings on the life course.

The emphasis on health in this argument is, however, relevant to gender and ageing. Following Gubrium's (1986) analysis of the 'discovery and conceptual elaboration' of Alzheimer's disease in the US, Featherstone and Hepworth argue that the establishment and redrawing of boundaries between normal and pathological ageing carry with them a powerful set of images of 'old age as a mask which conceals the essential identity of the person beneath' (1989: 148). The main idea here is that there is an essentially youthful person behind such masks, as people simultaneously embrace and deny the physiological ageing process. As older people become less marginalized and are drawn into mainstream culture, this may be at the expense of addressing questions brought about by inevitable biological limitations, disengagement and even death in later life.

As a dominant form of 'youthful' middle-aged (or populist Third Age) culture holds sway the message seems to be that we are all capable of being young now. This process may be particularly disadvantageous to older women, as youthful glamorous looks and sexuality are emphasized as positive attributes of this youthful culture. The implication remains that women's value is still strongly influenced by sexual attractiveness, and youthful appearance, in contrast to older men. It is little wonder that television sitcoms on later life in Britain and the US have recently given such poignant expression to the contradictions and dilemmas of such a situation.

Assessing the life approach

In summary, life course perspectives are emerging amongst the most widely used sociological approaches to age and ageing. Whether these are employed to explore the experiences of different age and social groups, or as a means of uncovering the 'cultural construction' of ageing, it is likely that variations of a life course perspective will continue to provide a dominant framework.

However, the life course perspective also faces some difficulties, particularly in a period in which the political agenda in many countries is characterized by 'chronic crises' in public spending and the restructuring of welfare. One of the most obvious criticisms against 'postmodern' theorizing is that such crises may exacerbate inequalities in old age, rather than ushering in a more pluralistic and non-hierarchical, let alone 'playful' scene (Fennell et al. 1988: 52).

There are now several examples of attempts to bring together elements of the 'political economy' approach and that of the life course, at least in the first strand identified above. Arber and Evandrou's (1993) approach notes the neglect of life course issues in official government thinking, and the potential impact that macro level policies, for example on social security, may have on matters such as patterns of care and disability across the life course. Recent discussions on restructuring in welfare states, and new models being developed to address it, have examined more explicitly the ways in which structured dependency is influenced by gender across the life course (e.g. Baldwin and Falkingham 1994).

There is a point here, though, that needs further consideration. Although a life course perspective constitutes a useful organizing framework for social research, it too often remains vague at a theoretical level. For example, though much of the work under discussion seems to revolve round trying to bring macro and micro levels together, the problems in doing so are not addressed in any depth. As a result, issues of agency and structure are touched upon, but little attempt is made to contribute explicitly to sociological theory. The problem with developing a life course approach in the absence of such theorizing is that it offers an overly 'horizontal' view of social life, characterized by transitions and change over time (meaning, variously, biographical and historical time) onto which material influences are seen to impinge. In fact, the sociological importance of these influences (or rules and resources) is that they are features of social hierarchies, which have implications for the distribution of power and status in everyday settings.

In other words, the links between macro and micro levels of analysis in the ageing field would be more clear *sociologically* if the contexts in which they occur were brought fully into focus. The outcomes or effects of disability and health status over time, for example, frequently depend on the macro level on government policies, and at the micro level on the character of institutional settings, such as clinics and social services departments. The exercise of power, and the counter-effects which social action might have on such hierarchies is critical to an understanding of ageing and the life course, particularly in a period of rapid change. Yet these processes are rarely discussed.

The experience of gender and ageing relates to more than the ability, in some general way, to mobilize resources. It is also a function of differences in power, within specific social hierarchies, which affect action. Thus attempts by people to cope with or undertake transitions may be cut across by their lack of power, or by the domination of one group over another, an issue which is rarely examined explicitly in research on ageing. Moreover, a rather rhetorical emphasis on meanings and 'everyday life', as being important features of ageing, may miss the point that 'less ordinary people' may exercise disproportionate influence over life chances (Mouzelis 1991:78). The actions and interests of the powerful, and the conflicts they engender, should feature more strongly in work on ageing. The postmodernist emphasis on 'de-hierarchicization' seems a particularly limited notion from this viewpoint.

In short, while the life course perspective is currently giving rise to a wave of new thinking and research on ageing, the theoretical basis of the approach remains underdeveloped. In particular, the interaction of class and gender in old age is weakly specified. Social inequalities *among* older people have thus been paradoxically obscured, as in the structured dependency argument, which emphasizes poverty as characteristic of old age. In turn, a close examination of the relationship between agency and structure in the life course approach has been largely ignored, partly as a result of an overreliance over on aggregate secondary data in much of the discussion of issues such as dependency and disability.

Among cultural theorists, putative changes, especially in the position of women, have not been examined critically, bearing in mind that negative images of women's roles persist. If the life course perspective is to be more sensitive to the experience of old age, clearer links need to be made between social circumstances and perceptions, and especially how far people identify with the changes in culture discussed here. More theoretically informed research is needed (including qualitative studies of particular localities) which examines the constraints in later life (especially those of class and gender) and the individual and collective strategies people devise to deal with them. In addition, more empirical evidence is needed on how far the supposed effect of a postmodern culture influences people's lives in different contexts. In this way the problem of agency and structure in old age may be given a clearer focus in life course work than it has to date.

Conclusion

The conclusion of this chapter is that to develop a more adequate sociological view of ageing and gender, a more explicit use of a conceptual framework emphasizing both *social hierarchy* and *human agency* is needed. The employment of such an approach would provide a more theoretically consistent way to examine linkages between micro and macro levels, and the gendered nature of social relations in ageing. Finally, a more consistent sociological perspective would also help reveal the importance of age and gender to change in late modern societies.

3

Theorizing Age and Gender Relations

Julie McMullin

Gender is now generally included in studies on the sociology of ageing, either implicitly or explicitly. Studies on older people tend to either examine men and women separately or include gender as a variable in the analysis (see for example, McDaniel 1986; Gee and Kimball 1987; Marshall 1987b; Connidis 1989). Indeed, old age is often viewed, at least demographically, as a women's issue (McDaniel 1986; Denton *et al.* 1987; Gee and Kimball 1987) and ageing generally affects men and women differently (Marshall 1987a; Levy 1988). In view of the growing recognition of the importance of gender in later life, the lack of theoretical development concerning the relationship between gender and ageing seems incomprehensible.

Although there are notable exceptions (see Riley 1987), gender and age relations have been overlooked by many mainstream sociological theorists, as noted by Arber and Ginn (1991a, 1991b). By 'mainstream' is meant the dominant theories in the sociological field, such as stratification theory in research on inequality and exchange theory in family research. Feminist and ageing scholars have sought to fill this gap by developing theories which take either gender relations or age relations into account. However, because feminist scholars generally do not consider age relations (see for example, Barrett 1980; Hartmann 1981; Hartsock 1983; Jaggar 1983; Acker 1988) and ageing theorists tend not to focus on gender relations (see for example, Walker 1981; Dannefer 1984; Kohli 1988; Minkler and Cole 1991; Elder and O'Rand 1995), the relationship between gender and age remains theoretically under-explored (Nett 1982; Reinharz 1986; Levy 1988; Arber and Ginn 1991b).

Some researchers on ageing have integrated a feminist perspective into their work by treating gender relations as fundamental to social organization rather than simply using gender as a variable in their analysis (Abu-Laban 1981; Burwell 1982, 1984; Hess 1985; McDaniel 1986, 1989; Gee and Kimball 1987; Quadagno 1988; Aronson 1990; 1992; Arber and Ginn 1991a; Blieszner 1993; Calasanti 1993; Palo Stoller 1993). Although this research provides a more accurate and comprehensive account of older age, a theoretical gap remains. Questions as to why and how gender and age influence social life and which of these is more fundamental require consideration. Should age and gender relations be considered separately or together? How do class and race/ethnic relations fit in? The common thread linking these questions and one reason they remain unaddressed is the fact that older women are the largest demographic group yet to attain theoretical status in sociology.

Gee and Kimball (1987: 10) agree that 'the general failure to incorporate women into mainstream theoretical perspectives on ageing is a reflection of our resistance to incorporate women into society and, hence, into sociological and psychological research.' This statement highlights two important issues. First, power imbalances shape theoretical construction; a group's place within the social structure influences the amount of theoretical attention they are afforded. Thus, because older women tend to occupy a position of lower social status, especially in economic terms (McDaniel 1986; Stone 1989; Arber and Ginn 1991a), than men of all ages and younger women (unless the latter are single mothers), they are given less theoretical attention.

Second, to 'incorporate older women' into mainstream theoretical perspectives on ageing has at least two meanings. In one sense, it implies 'adding on' consideration of gender without significantly changing existing theory. In another sense, it suggests combining the parts into an integrated whole, which would entail reformulating the theory. Theoretical construction about age and gender could therefore follow a number of different paths. There are three distinct paths within the 'add on' approach, each of which will be outlined. First, gender relations or age relations could be added on to mainstream sociological theories. Second, gender could be added on to sociological theories of ageing, referred to as 'gendered ageing theory'. Third, age relations could be added on to feminist theory, referred to as 'feminist ageing theory'. The chapter will then suggest an alternative path which involves a fully integrated approach, that is, the reformulation of sociological theory to take into account both age relations and gender relations. The appropriate choice among these approaches is not altogether clear and each may have its merits.

Drawing on research and theory from sociological, feminist and ageing domains, the implications of the 'add on' options are assessed in this chapter. The account of the literature presented here is not meant to be exhaustive but rather to provide an illustration of the state of theoretical developments regarding gender and age relations. Finally, noting the problems inherent in 'add on' approaches, a brief outline is given of how the rethinking of social class might proceed if age and gender relations were integrated.

Limiting this discussion to gender, age, and class relations neglects ethnic and race relations as well as other bases of differentiation among individuals which are central to social organization. Indeed, others have documented the importance of race and ethnicity (Askham *et al.* 1993; Vincent and Mucrovčić 1993) and disability (Zarb 1993) in later life. This chapter recognizes that small steps in theorizing about gender and age must be made before other aspects of differentiation and social organization can be considered.

In this chapter, use of the terms feminist theory, ageing theory, and sociological theory is not meant to imply that there is a single perspective in each of these branches of social theory (see Mike Bury's Chapter 2 for a discussion of the distinction between social and sociological theory). Rather, it is a way to classify theories according to their main focus. For example, the explicit emphasis in feminist theories on gender relations and women (usually younger women) is what groups these theories together. Likewise, at the core of ageing theories are issues associated with age relations and older adults. This chapter discusses the need for a sociological theory that explicitly considers age and gender relations simultaneously and with equal weight.

Which path is best travelled?

Adding gender and/or age to mainstream sociological theory

The practice of some theorists adding gender and others adding age to mainstream sociological theory has been prominent for many years, the assumption being that gender and age are characteristics that explain variance in a particular area of research. Although feminist scholars have been critical of this approach, ageing theorists have employed it. Indeed, one might easily confuse a survey of the social theories that have been put forward to explain the life situations of older people (Marshall 1987c; Fry 1992) with a survey of sociological theory in general. The same could not be said of feminist theories.

Feminist theorists have recognized that mainstream sociological theory is inadequate because it makes assumptions about the nature of paid work and home life that, although suitable to men, do not adequately represent the lives of women. Ageing theorists, on the other hand, have (with some notable exceptions) failed to question the assumptions underlying mainstream theories, examining the lives of older people within established sociological frameworks. The productive and reproductive lives of younger people are the ideal against which older people are judged. However, it cannot be assumed that mainstream theories about the nature of work and home life among young adults are appropriate for understanding the lives of older individuals. Some of the assumptions of family and stratification theory are briefly discussed; it is argued that the feminist critique of these theories is equally applicable to age relations.

Feminist theorists have been critical of mainstream theory on the family because it ignores issues such as gendered power imbalances and domestic labour which are salient to the lives of women. Many ageing theorists, on the other hand, accept the mainstream sociological evaluation of the traditional nuclear family. For example, it is often assumed that living within a nuclear family unit which functions as a 'haven' for its members and as a socialization agent for its children is ideal. This leads to a focus on the *problems* assumed to accompany deviation from this ideal as families age, such as the effect of the 'empty nest', changes in marital satisfaction and childlessness among older adults. It is assumed that the dynamics surrounding these issues are the same for younger and older individuals. However, recent research suggests that the 'empty nest' is welcomed by most couples (White and Edwards 1990) and that childlessness in older age is not necessarily problematic (Connidis and McMullin 1993). Nor is it clear that the factors contributing to marital satisfaction are the same for younger and older individuals (see Chapter 8 for further discussion). Thus family theories of ageing, because they incorporate assumptions from mainstream theory, fall prey to criticisms about age relations similar to those voiced by feminist scholars about gender relations. Approaches which simply add age to existing family theory neglect issues which are salient to older people, such as relationships with grandchildren, siblings and other extended family members, and the negotiation of leisure time within the context of family life. Feminists have attempted to rethink families by integrating issues which pervade the lives of women into their theories. Ageing theorists may learn from this and seek to rethink family theory, taking age relations specifically into account.

Feminists have been critical of the way mainstream stratification theories assess the economic situation of women by adding them on to existing theory. Ageing theorists, on the other hand, have employed these models within the dynamic of a life course perspective to explain income differentials among those who are no longer employed. The premise in this school of thought is that previous position in the labour market strongly influences one's social status in later life. Kohli (1988: 376) points to potential problems with this approach. First, social status in later life, although it is related to earlier employment, is also influenced by other factors. Second, some stratification models assess rank among older people as a whole, ignoring the inequalities between age groups. Third, this approach rarely considers the relational aspects of class associated with control and subordination. Models based on individual achievement (e.g. education) and job characteristics (e.g. unionization, job tenure) are far less useful in explaining income inequality among older people than younger, suggesting that for older people other factors become more pertinent to their economic situation (McMullin and Ballantyne 1994). Thus there is something unique about age relations that is inadequately represented in stratification models designed to differentiate among younger people.

In sum, the central problems associated with adding gender or age on to mainstream sociological theories are as follows. First, in these paradigms, social life is assumed to vary according to the particular characteristic that is to be added to an established theory. In other words, rather than treating social life as organized and structured around a particular set of relations, like age relations, these theories simply use age as a variable that is the basis of difference. Next, the emphasis on difference necessarily assumes an ideal referent, most often a white middle-class male, from which others deviate according to characteristics such as gender and age. The third assumption implicit in 'adding on' gender or age is that the categories established to study the reference group are suitable for all groups. For example, 'family' is assumed to be an appropriate construct with suitable categories for the study of older people and women. The feminist critique of mainstream sociological theory shows that these points of contention are not new (see Acker 1980, 1988; Fox 1989; Calasanti and Zajicek 1993). However, their application to theorizing about age and the intersection between age and gender relations may provide new insights regarding the possibility of adding gender to ageing theory or age to feminist theory (see Calasanti and Zajicek 1993).

Adding gender to sociological theories of ageing

For the purpose of this chapter, 'sociological theories of ageing' refer to theories that have gone beyond adding age on to sociological theory and instead have reconceptualized age relations. Although open to criticism, notable examples of these theories include modernization theory (Cowgill and Holmes 1972), several versions of the political economy of ageing (Walker 1981; Estes, *et al.* 1982; Estes 1983; Guillemard 1983; Myles 1989), and the recent calls for and theoretical development of critical theory (Kohli *et al.* 1983; Moody 1988; Baars 1991; Minkler and Estes 1991). In general, these theories have either ignored gender or have noted the importance of gender relations but have lacked any theoretical development.

The recognition of gender points to the value of developing what is referred to here as gendered ageing theory. It is necessary, however, to consider whether the sociological understanding of later life would be strengthened by adding gender relations on to ageing theory and how this theoretical development would take shape within ageing frameworks.

If the inclusion of gender in theories of ageing is to improve our understanding of the social lives of older individuals, the life situations of older women and men would have to be influenced by different factors. If they are not, then it would be unnecessary to consider gender relations in theories regarding age relations. Although it is clear that the socioeconomic and family situations of men and women in later life are different (Kendig 1986; McDaniel 1986; Mugford and Kendig 1986; Gee and Kimball 1987; Marshall 1987b; Chapman 1989; Connidis 1989; Arber and Ginn 1991a), such divergence does not in itself warrant distinct theory. Rather, the factors contributing to variation must also be different in order to justify separate theoretical consideration.

Gerontological research shows that men and women follow different life-course paths leading to variations in economic well-being and family resources throughout later life. For instance, because women tend to be financially dependent on men, have more irregular work histories, and live longer than men, they have smaller pensions and are more likely than their male counterparts to exhaust their financial resources in later life; their economic well-being in later life is influenced by their marital status in a way that men's is not (Arber and Ginn 1991a). Thus women are more likely than men to experience poverty for the *first* time in later life. On the other hand, men are more likely to maintain the same relative social class in older age as they had when they were younger (McDaniel 1986, 1989). With regard to family (but not economic) status, divorce generally has a greater negative impact on the family relations of older men than of older women (Mugford and Kendig 1986; Chapman 1989). This suggests that there are gender differences in the factors that contribute to the maintenance of family relationships in later life.

However, adding gender relations to ageing theory is limiting because other factors that contribute to the life worlds of men and women are often not considered. For instance, ageing theorists' tendency to neglect domestic labour relations or gendered power imbalances in their assessment of class or family relations demonstrates the limitations of taking this theoretical direction.

How then, would this theoretical development take place? Based on the assumptions of 'add on' approaches it is likely that, implicit in the construction of gendered ageing theory there would be an emphasis on age relations over and above gender relations. The categories of analysis would necessarily be those that are already established within the confines of the theories mentioned above and gender would have to be dealt with according to those frameworks.

Like mainstream sociological theorists, ageing theorists often assume that white middle-class young men are the referent with which other social groups should be compared. Adding women and gender differences into these theories is likely to result in older men being the ideal to which older women are compared. Researchers tend either to treat gender as a variable in the analysis, comparing one sex to the other or to separate men and women and assume that the same categories of analysis are appropriate for both (Calasanti and Zajicek 1993).

In the theoretical arena, political economy approaches appear to follow this path of including women but without rethinking existing models. For example, according to Walker (1981: 76), inequality in later life is related to 'employment status and socio-economic group prior to retirement, which in turn rests partly on social class of origin'. He goes on to suggest that unequal access to occupational pensions is based primarily on socioeconomic group, employment status, and historical changes in pension conditions. Recognizing that, as a group, older women are among the most economically disadvantaged, Walker (1981: 87) adds women on to his model by describing their situation as primarily a result of 'segregative employment policies, discriminatory social policies restricting access to resources on an equal basis to men,

[and] depressed social status relative to men, which disadvantage them during their working lives'. Walker makes the uncritical assumption that traditional conceptualizations of constructs such as 'social class' and 'socio-economic group' are appropriate in understanding the poverty of older women. Although occupational class explains much of the income inequality among older people, for women marital status and childbearing history are equally important (Ginn and Arber 1991, 1993). Further, how and why processes such as segregative employment policies are put into place are not considered. Nor are other aspects of gender inequality such as access to leisure time and divisions of household labour considered. A final problem, in this and other political economy approaches (Estes *et al.* 1982; Estes 1983; Guillemard 1983; Myles 1989), is discussed by Mike Bury in Chapter 2. As he argues, the emphasis on social structure in these theories leads to a failure to consider the way in which gendered hierarchies are shaped by cultural factors and by individual and collective agency as well as by macro level processes.

This section has demonstrated that a better sociological understanding of later life requires the consideration of gender relations. Further, although adding gender on to ageing research and theory is a positive step, this approach is inadequate to explain the economic and family situations of older women (see also Hendricks 1993).

Adding age relations on to feminist theory

The final 'add on' approach considered is adding age on to feminist theory. If a feminist ageing theory is to be justified, current feminist theory must be deficient in explaining the life-worlds of older women. In other words, if there is nothing distinctive about being an older woman, beyond just being a woman and just being older, then feminist ageing theory is not required. Age and gender must be multiplicative in their effect on economic and family situations if feminist ageing theory is to enhance our understanding of older women in society.

Some insight may be gained from the concept of double jeopardy. The double jeopardy (or double whammy) hypothesis, as it applies to older women, posits that older women are at a heightened disadvantage due to both their gender and their age (Posner 1977; Chappell and Havens 1980). Research has shown that older women are at greater risk of experiencing mental health problems, poverty, disability and age discrimination, than younger adults and older men (Posner 1977; Chappell and Havens 1980; McDaniel 1986; Gee and Kimball 1987; Arber and Ginn 1991a). These findings suggest that there is something distinctive about being an older woman. Furthermore, as the preceding section demonstrates, the factors that contribute to the life-worlds of older women are different from those of older men. The gendered nature of domestic labour, discrimination and oppression in the workplace, power imbalances within the family, and the changing age relations that surround these issues through the life course, have all contributed to the lives of older women. In order to understand gender relations among older adults these issues must be considered and feminist theory provides a means of doing so. However, there is a risk that age relations will take second place to gender if age is added on to feminist theory. In this case, the categories and frameworks used by feminist theorists would be applied to age. It is illuminating to consider some examples of research using this approach.

The paradigms employed in some of the research on caregiving are illustrative of a feminist approach to an age-related issue (Finley 1989; Aronson 1990; 1992). Thus, using theories of family labour to assess gender differences in caregiving for elderly parents, Finley (1989) concludes that these theories do not adequately explain women's higher commitment than men's to caring for their older parents. Rather, gender relations structure the nature of caregiving and regardless of time availability, relative power, specialization of tasks or gender socialization, women assume responsibility for care (see also Aronson 1992). Recognizing, however, the potential power imbalances which are shaped by age relations in caregiving situations, it is evident that what these accounts lack is an explicit examination of the intersection of age relations with the gendered relations of care. Similarly, where researchers have used a socialist feminist approach to issues pertinent to older people, such as retirement, lay health care, and widowhood (Blieszner 1993; Calasanti 1993; Palo Stoller 1993), the intersections among gender, race and class relations have tended to take precedence over age relations. These researchers (for example Calasanti and Zajicek 1993) agree with Hess (1990) in assuming that inequalities between the sexes in old age 'are not unique to that life stage but are continuous, with patterned inequalities throughout the life course' (Hess 1990: 12). However, we must recognize that these inequalities are *both* patterned throughout the life course and are related to age (see double jeopardy research above and Kohli 1988). In other words, potential power imbalances which are structured by age relations must also be considered.

Towards a gender and age relations theory

The difficulties inherent in each of these 'add on' theoretical approaches can be resolved by recognizing that age and gender relations cannot be treated as separate systems which shape life situations. If age and gender are organizing dimensions of the social world, then separating these systems makes no sense. Older people are not just old, they are either men or women. As sociologists studying ageing, we do not view our subjects as simply men or women but as older men and older women. Although this point may seem obvious and even simplistic, it is not translated into theory and only rarely is it recognized in research (see Aronson 1990; Arber and Ginn 1991a; for research examples). The debate among feminist theorists as to whether the two systems that operate to oppress women – patriarchy and capitalism – can be theoretically treated as separate is relevant here. Just as it is inappropriate to separate patriarchy from capitalism because the two systems do not operate in isolation from each another (see Fox 1988), the separation of age and gender relations is also problematic.

The difficulty lies in knowing how to proceed but a first step is to reconceptualize the categories of social analysis. For instance, if social inequality is the object of theory, it is unlikely that gender and age relations can be adequately explained within current social class frameworks. Instead, social class must be rethought, placing less emphasis on the traditional Marxist or Weberian conceptualizations. This is not to say that all theory as it stands now should be abandoned. Rather, that theory must be reformulated instead of expanded. Although the rest of this chapter will be devoted to a discussion of social inequality, this point is equally relevant in other areas of research. Indeed, Terri Whittaker, in writing about gender and elder abuse (Chapter 11) makes a similar point by suggesting that the methodological problems in this field stem from an attempt to fit elder abuse into 'malestream' frameworks of individual or family pathology.

Although it is beyond the scope of this chapter to embark on a major development of theory, Acker's (1988) work on the relations of distribution in the conceptualization of social class will be used to illustrate how such rethinking might proceed. Although Acker does not consider age relations, her attempt at integrating gender and class provides a theoretical model to guide the rethinking of the intersections between age, gender and class. Taking issue with dual systems theory (that capitalism and patriarchy are separate but interacting systems; Hartmann 1981; Walby 1986), Acker (1988) sets out to develop a single system theory of social relations that places equal emphasis on gender and class. According to Acker this requires a reformulation of Marx's conception of class, in which the social relations of distribution as well as production are taken into account.

Acker suggests that the wage is the essential component of distribution in capitalist society. Because women have always been paid less than men and gendered job segregation is pervasive, the wage has developed historically as a gendered phenomenon. Personal relations, marital relations, and state relations are the gendered processes through which distribution occurs. Personal relations of distribution are held together by emotional bonds, usually between blood relatives, and are dependent upon the wage. Marital relations are of key importance, because married women who do not work for pay are dependent upon their husbands for economic support. Thus, according to Acker, unwaged housewives are connected to the production process through their husbands' wages. Although they share common standards of living with their husbands they do not share the same class because their situations, experiences and activities are different. Unwaged wives have little control over their economic situation although this may vary according to the man's and woman's class. State relations of distribution take over when there is no wage or it is inadequate. The wage labour system is influenced by the state through legislative measures that affect men, women and minority groups differently (for example, legislation on pensions, disability and unemployment benefits, wage supplements and redundancy payments). Hence, class is structured through the gendered relations of distribution and production (Acker 1988: 495).

It is worth considering briefly how Acker's thesis could be enhanced if age relations were integrated into the theory. Acker (1988) suggests that in all known societies the relations of distribution and production are influenced by gender and thus take on gendered meaning. Gender relations of distribution in capitalist society are historically rooted and are transformed as the means of production change. The same could be said for age relations. For instance, although it was rare to live to be very old in agricultural societies, those who did so would at least partially retire from farming and would have to rely on their children to distribute enough food and resources to them for their subsistence (Mitterauer and Sieder 1982). A Hindu sage, Manu, propounded a doctrine dictating the rules of withdrawal from society that a man should follow if he 'sees his skin wrinkled, and his hair white, and the sons of his sons' (McKee 1982: 14). According to Manu, older men should be supported through alms and afforded the luxury of not having to be concerned with practical matters of survival (McKee 1982). (It is perhaps significant that Manu made no recommendations as to how older women should be supported.) Thus the relations of distribution in these societies are structured by age relations.

In capitalist society as well, age relations are fundamental to the relations of distribution. Wages, the essential component of distribution in capitalist society, take on a specific meaning depending on age and indeed have developed historically as an age-related phenomenon. Today, teenagers work for less money than young adults, who in turn work for less money than middle-aged adults and these trends are structured according to the gender relations outlined by Acker. Thus in the present capitalist system, it is the intersection between age-related and gendered processes that structure the wage distribution which is an important factor (along with wealth, power, autonomy, and ownership of the means of production, which Acker does not consider) in assessing social class.

Young children rely on their personal relations with their parents for the distribution of adequate resources. Many older people rely on resources distributed by the state or, less often, from their children. Marital relations of distribution take on a different meaning in widowhood, as the remaining spouse has a legal entitlement to assets and often to benefits from occupational pensions. Women are far more likely to be widowed and also to inherit assets and income from their spouse than men. Thus the influence of age in the processes that shape the relations of production and distribution are clear. That gender relations intersect in each of these processes simultaneously is also evident.

To summarize, social class is structured through age-based and gendered relations of distribution and production. The links between class, gender, and age are best understood if class is rethought to include both the relations of production and of distribution. Thus the analysis of social inequality must consider the interacting influence of gender and age relations and must do so through a reformulation of social class that takes distribution into account.

The point of this discussion is to demonstrate how the rethinking of a social theory, which already considers gender and class relations, might proceed if age relations were taken into account. The strength of Acker's argument lies in its conceptualization of a class system which includes individuals who are not employed in the paid labour force. This point alone renders the theory particularly useful to those who are interested in understanding age relations. However, there are several problems with Acker's theory and its rethinking that require attention. First, although it is true that there has always been a division of labour based on sex and age, there is evidence which suggests that these divisions do not always translate into inequality (Coontz and Henderson 1986). Thus, it is not clear how the processes of distribution and production became unequally structured by gender and age prior to the development of feudal and capitalist societies.

Second, in rethinking Marx's conceptualization of class, Acker limits her discussion to the structural aspects of social inequality. This approach ignores cultural dimensions of inequality and how these influence gender and age-based social hierarchies (see Mike Bury's Chapter 2). Related to this are the neglected questions of personal and collective agency and the means by which individuals and groups strive for power while being confined by limited choices available to them. Finally, it may be problematic to restrict the discussion of social inequality to the distribution of money (Taylor and Ford 1983). Broadening this discussion to include other potential sources of inequality such as health and psychological functioning, social support (Taylor and Ford 1983), differences in leisure time and activity, and inequality in the division of household labour may prove fruitful in theoretical construction.

Summary and conclusions

The aim of this chapter is to demonstrate the need for comprehensive theories of gender and age relations and to provide insight into the directions this theorizing could take. 'Add on' approaches tend to focus on the difference that gender and age make in relation to a particular area of study rather than recognizing that social life is organized around gender and age relations as well as the relations of class and race. Thus, a central goal in 'add on' approaches is to compare women to men, and older to younger people, with men and the young often serving as ideal referents. However, if gender and age relations simultaneously structure social life, examining differences between these groups is like comparing apples and oranges. Gender and age relations also interact with class and race relations in the structuring of social life. The limited evidence offered in this chapter on the age and gendered processes that shape individual lives provides indirect justification for assuming interaction among these four dimensions.

'Add on' approaches also assume that the categories of investigation are suitable for all groups of people. However, as Acker (1988) shows, relations of production are inadequate for assigning class to women. Thus theory has to be rethought and categories reconceptualized in order to achieve a better understanding of the situation of older people in general and older women in particular. Using Acker's (1988) theory of the relations of distribution is one way in which this rethinking could take place. Social class has to be reconceptualized by thinking about the age and gendered processes that influence the relations of distribution and production. This represents only one possible solution to the problem and the relative simplicity of this discussion should not be interpreted as underestimating the complexity of the task. Instead, this discussion could serve as a starting point from which feminist and ageing theorists could launch new ideas and theories that would improve our understanding of the social lives of older women and men. Further, it could stimulate new sociological theory on social inequality and social class.

In future theoretical development, macro level issues concerning the nature of the relationship between gender and age-based systems of inequality and capitalism are central, as is the case in political economy approaches. However, it is important also to consider the relationship between social structure and cultural factors and how human agency plays a role in determining social status. Finally, the construct of social inequality should be broadened to include a range of other personal resources.

Acknowledgements

I am grateful to several scholars who have provided comments on earlier versions of this chapter and who have talked over gender and age relations with me. These include: Sara Arber, Peri Ballantyne, Ingrid Connidis, Lorraine Davies, Bonnie Fox, Jay Ginn and Victor Marshall. My work on this project has been supported by a Social Science and Humanities Research Council Scholarship, the Donald Menzies–CAG Bursary, and the Naomi Grigg Fellowship in Gerontology.

4

CONFORMITY AND RESISTANCE AS WOMEN AGE

Doris Ingrisch

The contradictions between women's socially prescribed roles and the reality of their daily lives have been explored in women's studies. The conflicts of women who want to have both a career and to fulfil their duties according to the traditional sequential roles of the virgin, the sexually desirable object, and the 'good mother' have been documented. These studies, however, are largely limited to women under 60 years of age; the older woman is either not included at all or is treated as of peripheral importance, as noted by Peace (1986) and Arber and Ginn (1991b).

In this chapter, older women are brought centre stage and given a voice through their life histories. Thirty life history interviews were collected in a study conducted for the Austrian Ministry of Women's Affairs and the Society of Ageing and Culture in Vienna. The study centred on socially transmitted images of women's roles and how these images were related to age and identity (Anderson and Ingrisch 1992). The older women's lives are also related to the historical context in which they lived: a central European country, Austria, which underwent changes from a monarchy at the beginning of the century to a republic, followed by a fascist regime and, after World War II, a republic again.

In the study, the intention was to allow theoretical ideas to emerge through analysing and interpreting the women's accounts, rather than approaching the interviews with a particular theoretical orientation. The analysis of life histories is recommended by Fuchs (1984: 197) as facilitating a comprehensive and interdisciplinary view of social life: 'using the perspective of a biography enables a global and complex ... view of the social environment to be achieved'. An approach which gives priority to subjects' own accounts may be especially valuable in researching women's lives:

> In contrast to a theoretical construction of the world, research in women's and gender studies brings together folklore and historical research about day-to-day life. It leaves theory aside . . . and attempts to reconstruct the informal logic of life.
>
> (Lipp 1988: 32)

In the following biographical accounts, an attempt is made both to give women a voice and to use the researchers' own experiences to interpret their meaning, 'for when we interpret, we bring our knowledge, experience, and concerns to our material, and the result, we hope, is a richer, more textured understanding . . .' (Borland 1991: 73).

In all of the 30 interviews, two levels of experience were apparent. The first level represents conformity to society's expectations; in the women's own words, they 'do the right thing', thinking and behaving in terms of clearly defined social roles. The second level is concerned with suppressed wishes and longings, which may be understood as the level of 'authenticity'. The conflicts and contradictions expressed by women in their life histories demonstrate their efforts to find a balance between the outer and the inner world – between society's expectations and their own aspirations. Women quite often tried to evade these conflicts and adapt to society's standards, taking on the roles of the 'good mother', 'good grandmother', or the 'perfect daughter'. Because of the importance of these prescribed gender roles in stabilizing social systems, questions arise as to how they are changing and the social consequences of these changes.

The life stories of three older women are used in this chapter as exemplars, to illustrate some of the ways in which older women had dealt with conflicts arising from gender roles. The three cases have been selected to reflect special aspects of the biographies collected. They exemplify how patterns of tension between social norms and individual lives change with succeeding generations. Although all three women came from bourgeois families in Vienna, they differed in important ways: in how they managed their own lives in the context of specific historical periods; in what they emphasized as their identity within the interviews; in the kind of conflicts they faced; and finally, in the strategies they used to resolve conflicts.

Two of the women were born in 1914, at the start of World War I. They have therefore lived through two world wars and were children in the 1920s, when the 'new woman' appeared on the societal stage: emancipated and insolent. As young women they lived in a political climate first of Austro-fascism and then of National Socialism. This is a period most of the women avoided mentioning. A strong taboo discourages discussion of these years, especially when people are confronted with their own political responsibility. However, the few things the women did mention in their interviews give insight into their understanding of women's roles during these years. When the second-wave feminist movement started in Austria these women were almost 60 years old and they were aged 78 at the time of interview. The third woman, 14 years younger, was born in 1928. In her 40s, she was surrounded by the revolutionary social movements of the 1970s which initiated new visions in society, especially of women's roles and rights. At that time women in Austria also became more active in public affairs, published magazines and papers in support of individual rights and systematically questioned traditional gender patterns. Because of her later birth, the third woman – representing a later generation – experienced the changing social and political trends at a younger age than the first two women.

First case: Ms U

Background

Ms U was born in 1914 in Vienna, where she attended primary and secondary school. Before taking the secondary school final exams, she began to work part time at the company where her father was employed. Starting as a telephonist, she quickly worked her way up to administrative secretary, as she proudly related. She got married but soon lost her husband in World War II. As a result of the political upheavals in 1938, Ms U left the company and then worked in a military factory in the mineral oil branch. In 1942 her services were required in the aircraft division and she worked as a secretary in a highly confidential position. When the staff fled to the West in March 1945, she remained with her parents in their bombed out apartment, hoping her husband would return from the front. However, he did not return.

After a time, she found work again and met her second husband, whom she married in 1950. One year later she gave birth to a son. She worked in her husband's grocery store for 15 years until she had to sell it due to her husband's serious illness. For the 11 years until her retirement she had a job in an office. At the time of the interview, which took place in her apartment, Ms U was serving as Honorary District Director of the Conservative Party. Ms U was trim and tastefully dressed in a skirt and blouse and gave a lively and friendly impression. She showed me her school reports and family photographs and enjoyed talking about herself and her life.

Analysis and interpretation

Ms U described her mother and father as being 'the best parents one could possibly imagine'. When her father returned from the war in 1919, he took over her upbringing. 'My mother never interfered in the child rearing, that was my father's job' and she learned to interpret 'always being there' as love. Anything other than a loving father would not have fitted her image of a happy family. However, she also says: 'he was quick to give me spankings . . . or make me kneel in the corner . . . but maybe I had deserved it'. When she begins to tell of her puberty, she almost speaks in her father's voice: 'I became very reasonable and understood that one wasn't allowed to do this or one wasn't allowed to do that'. Her use of the word 'one' in this context suggests that she is referring to societal norms represented by her father's rules. Her 'insight' then is the recognition of society's expectations. Her own perception had apparently been totally blacked out. She was beginning to internalize what constituted 'doing the right thing'.

Her 'first true love' was a man whom she described as comical. Her mother recognized in this dapper young man someone who could take over her daughter's 'further' education, in terms of conforming to her feminine role as a wife. She encouraged her daughter to marry him, which she did. Like many relationships of this generation, this one was destroyed by World War II. When Ms U's husband did not return from the war, it was her father who at first consoled her and then encouraged her to start looking for another husband. She followed his advice without even considering her own wishes. 'And then I got married for the second time in 1950, although I hadn't had the slightest intention of getting married again.' 'I thought about my dead husband all the time and cried constantly', she remembered. Even though she wasn't in love with her new husband – he had fallen in love with her, but not vice versa – and her own preference had been not to remarry, she still did what was expected of her. She tried to 'do the right thing' and justified her action as a 'good deed'. While her first marriage fitted both her own desires and her expected gender role, the second marriage, brought about indirectly by National Socialism and the war, was not anticipated and created a dilemma. She found that embracing religious ideals offered her a way out, by distancing her from real life and by elevating her to the status of a 'saint'.

Ms U became pregnant shortly after the wedding – again conforming to 'the right thing'. Although her pregnancy improved her relationship with her second husband, she found the condition 'distasteful' and the bodily processes unpleasant; the birth itself, which she referred to as a 'business', she found particularly so. The new baby enriched her life, especially through the constant confirmation that she was needed. 'The relationship with dolls and little children was always enormously satisfying for me. Also with animals, cats, dogs, everything that was helpless', she explained, justifying her enthusiasm about the role of mother and nurse. In bringing up her son, she resumed the behavioural pattern of 'always being there' that she had learned in childhood from her father as the meaning of love. 'There was only one single occasion when my baby wore an un-ironed diaper,' she recalled. 'I was an enthusiastic mother. That baby was a "holy relic" for me.' The style and content of her language point again to a strong religious influence upon her concept of the world. When asked about her religious beliefs, she spoke of the image most important to her, that of Mary, the mother of God. The Madonna represents the benevolent self-sacrificing saint, an image which, especially in Catholic countries like Austria, served and still serves as a cultural role model.

In spite of her dedication to the mother role, combining work outside the home with motherhood did not trouble her at all; to be successful at both was proof of her willingness for self-sacrifice. Ms U was extremely proud that she had worked alongside her father in the factory as a young woman and later, as a mother, had helped in her husband's business. 'I wasn't unemployed for one single hour, for the reason that I was such a decent and conscientious worker, perhaps a bit too decent and conscientious, that no one had a thing to complain about.' In her working life, she saw herself as a woman who would 'do the right thing', in terms of what others — society — expected of her. Only once did she wonder if she had been too compliant, by articulating the notion of being 'too decent'. Her strategy for dealing with this was to shift her overconformity into the moral domain; she had just been 'too' good, 'too' decent. It was in connection with this idea of overconscientiousness that she mentioned her position of trust in the wartime factory. In her working life, as in her home life, her need to be needed by others was dominant.

The year 1976 must have been one of the most difficult for Ms U. Both professionally and privately her 'reason for being' — to work for others and to be irreplaceable — was suddenly pulled out from under her feet. She felt she was no longer needed. 'Although I had always had a lot to do, and sometimes didn't know if I was coming or going, I was still taken by surprise when I was suddenly without an occupation; my retirement, the death of my husband, and my son's moving out, being the final separation.' Because other people were essential to her definition of herself and her roles, the loss of the familiar structure led her into a serious crisis.

Her condition did not stabilize until her family — the decisive authority for women who have internalized the classic gender roles — once again satisfied her 'need to be needed'. With the magic words: 'Mummy, we need you', Ms U was again confirmed in her reason for being. She said proudly: 'Since that time . . . I have always been surrounded by family; my children [her son and daughter-in-law] live in the same house, we have the best relationship imaginable, there is no generation gap, everything is right'. Again everything seemed just as it should be. Since being needed was important to her, getting older, in the sense of not being needed, was threatening. To be in need of help herself or inactive was what most frightened her about ageing. So far she had managed to avoid this, and in this instance her mother served as her role model. 'I do everything myself, I don't receive help for anything, and my apartment is certainly not untidy. I also take care of my body, my mother did just the same.' Because her happiness depended on the happiness of others and because order represented the most important demand in her life, she felt no other desires and was probably correct in affirming: 'I am not unhappy.'

For Ms U, getting older did not bring liberation from societal constraints, but rather anxiety due to loss of her previous roles. It was possible, however, for her to slip into a new role, that of the wise old woman. As an authoritative mother to her own child, she was able to continue this role in giving advice to young women. Referring to a fellow member in the Conservative Party, Ms U said, 'She is a very young woman, and actually takes me seriously, follows all the advice that I give her. And it is certainly worth a lot to me that I can still be of help to young people.' She presented herself as an understanding and motherly woman who could draw from a wealth of life experiences. With this ability, she remained in command. Because she defined herself so totally through the eyes of others, her self-esteem constantly depended on how much attention others paid her. Through authoritative behaviour, she was able to force others to pay her respect. Her son, and the young woman she referred to, were expected automatically to respect her because of her age and her role as the wise old mother. Ms U sought contact not only with younger people but also with older ones, most of them women. The fact that these relationships were part of an age-hierarchal power structure was revealed in her remarks about a friend who was 10 years older: 'She is always pleased when she is allowed to visit.' By using the word 'allow', Ms U demonstrates the power that younger adults have over older in later life.

Ms U embodies the type of woman who orients herself towards gendered social role images; she felt no need to search for an authentic self outside traditional feminine and work roles and never broke out of these designated roles. None of her remarks pointed to conflicts with socially defined role images. She emphasized many times that 'everything was in order'. But is it really *her* order? She appears to have clung to socially prescribed role images in order to transform her weaknesses into strengths. In order to live this out fully, she, in turn, had to oppress others, for example in the domineering way she dealt with her son or the young woman. Her eagerness to 'do the right thing', as recognized and accepted by society, helped to transmit traditional gender role images to the next generation.

In contrast, the next case considered represents those who experience conflicts over conforming to traditional gender roles, due to the rigidly gender-differentiated social environment.

Second case: Ms M

Background

Ms M was born in Vienna in 1914 as an only child in a family of teachers. She attended primary, then secondary school and enrolled at university to study gymnastics and French. In the autumn of 1939 she completed her university studies and immediately obtained a teaching post at a secondary school. In March 1945, she was granted membership of the National Socialist Party, an act which soon led to the termination of her teaching post, since at the end of the war all party members were suspended from civil service posts. In 1949 she was – like many others – reinstated and from that time until 1974 she remained at the same school. During the war, she married a colleague, who was killed in action a few months before the birth of their son. She lived on with her parents and later, for 15 years, took over the care of her father, when he was crippled following a stroke.

During the interview, Ms M's demeanour remained reserved and distant. The conversation took place in her apartment, which was furnished with Persian rugs, a grand piano and oil paintings, and which was located in an upper-middle-class neighbourhood. Ms M wore no make-up and was very modestly dressed in trousers and a jumper.

Analysis and interpretation

As Ms M spoke of her childhood, two main topics that she remembered clearly came into the conversation: her father and school. For example, 'My childhood was wonderful; my father was a teacher and a born pedagogue and knew exactly how to get along with children . . . we were a model class.'

When encouraged to talk about her career development, she began by expressing her pride in her father: 'everything that I know, and I know a lot about plants and animals, I learned from him'. Although her mother was also a teacher, as emerged later in the conversation, she repeated that *he* had been the cause of her choosing the teaching profession. Ms M portrayed her mother, with whom she had much in common – 'My mother was just as temperamental as I am' – as a nagging person with whom she had many disputes. 'I never felt put under pressure by my father, more so by my mother because she verbally insulted me.' She recalled the screaming contests she had with her mother, which she still could not explain except as stemming from the close similarity between herself and her mother.

As a teenager, the search for her role in life had caused many disturbances, which she excused as adolescent behaviour. For some rebellion 'is allowed' at this age; it is almost 'the right thing to do'. Because of the relative licence allowed in adolescence, serious conflicts over the sexual stereotypes and sex role guidelines of adult society are obscured.

In adulthood, the dilemma for Ms M of whether to identify with the masculine role model represented by the father she admired or with the feminine role model of her mother was only settled when her mother took on the traditional domestic role again in the family; while her mother kept house, as well as taking care of Ms M's son, Ms M herself to a large extent remained free. As a result she was able to reject much of the classical feminine role at that stage in her life.

For a young woman of her bourgeois social status, it was absolutely clear that she was expected to marry and have children. She did not dispute these societal expectations at the time. However, as she began to talk about her first encounter with her husband, she sounded very distant. Her description of the relationship was meagre, summed up by a cliché, and she soon shifted the focus by commenting on the quality of her relationship with her in-laws: 'I met him at university and, you know the saying, it was love at first sight. There were no substantial difficulties, even with my in-laws, who took to me instantly.' The fact that she continued to have rows with her husband, just as she had had with her mother, suggests there were similar conflicts over the determination of roles. Her husband may have wanted to define her in a stereotypical woman's role which she found unacceptable but was unable to discuss with him. She was clearly under stress at the time, which could be read as frustration at the powerlessness of women in society, which she refused to accept, as well as resistance to the power of the male patriarchy, which at the same time attracted her.

Ms M barely mentioned her son. In her description of him she only mentioned the key dates of his life, including his educational history, which she seemed to feel was especially worth mentioning. She did not say a word about the feelings she had for her son, whom she referred to, curiously, as 'the child' throughout the interview. What she did describe with great emotion was neither her child nor her role as mother, but the modified daughter role she played when she lived with her parents and the 15 years of caring for her father. After the death of her husband, at which time she was still a young woman, her father was the only man of importance in her life. She described it thus: 'I was a very childlike creature, that had very little interest in men and also had no relationship with men.' She used her father's need for her care as the reason, which can be interpreted as an excuse, for not getting involved in a relationship. 'Then there was my father, as I said, who had had a stroke, and getting married was just out of the question.' It seems as if Ms M had completely submerged the possibilities her own life had to offer, by accommodating her father's personality and needs. She learned to keep any feelings she had at bay. 'No, my life didn't change at all, it was always quite normal.'

Stuck in the role of the daughter, Ms M seems to have reached a compromise between her feminine and masculine sides. As well as being a dutiful daughter, it was also 'the right thing' to learn a trade. She described her choice of profession in a pragmatic manner: 'I enjoyed sports very much, so naturally I considered gymnastics; I had had eight years of French, so that possibility was open to me as well.' She displayed the same detached attitude in explaining what her profession had meant to her: 'In the last years of teaching I looked forward to my retirement, but otherwise I was able to come to terms with my job.' In teaching – one of the first middle-class professions open to women – she could manage very well; it offered her economic independence, while at the same time giving her sufficient freedom to care for her child and later for her sick father, exactly as she was expected to do. According to social norms at that time, this role combination was acceptable, while just a few decades earlier the role of mother had been denied to teachers, who were expected to remain celibate. She was thus able to live out a part of her masculine identification without any feelings of guilt about her career while at the same time she could fulfil familial duties within her feminine role. Having both these gender roles enabled her to care for her father, as she wished, but to delegate other typically feminine duties, when she found these too unpleasant. 'I liked to cook, but I let the others do the housework, something I still don't like to do to this day.' A career also served to stabilize her life. Her job and the demands it made on her provided her life with a firm structure to which she could orient herself and something to hold on to in difficult times. This is illustrated in her attitude to the death of her husband: 'Well, I felt somewhat like a schizophrenic. I immediately went back to work, if only to keep from thinking about it . . . I felt as if I was walking in a fog if I wasn't teaching at that very moment.'

After Ms M retired, the stabilizing influence of her employment was lost but the change offered her other ways to meet her needs. Retirement for Ms M, as for most of the women that were interviewed, was not nearly as difficult as the 'retirement shock' often said to be experienced by men. Once excused, or liberated, from many of her roles, that of the career woman, the educator, the mother and the nurse, she was able to do much more of what she enjoyed in her youth, namely sports, which she enjoyed more in later life than ever before. At the time of interview, she still played tennis three times a week. In addition, the club atmosphere kept her from feeling lonely. She had also retained her love of music, originally inspired, as she said, by her father. Thus the ending of her career was not at all difficult for her. She could now, in pursuing her hobbies, do what she enjoyed most. She could be herself, guided by her own standards rather than conforming to a certain gender role and, to some extent, be 'authentic'.

As a practical person, she had largely blocked out all fantasies and feelings. In order to avoid being drawn into conflicts, she developed the traditional masculine characteristics of denial of emotions and concentration on the 'facts'; in other words an adherence to rationality. She did not allow herself to feel sad or depressed, except of course when it was 'the right thing to do'. Ms M's choice of words can be used to infer a reference to social norms of behaviour. The German word 'man' (meaning 'one') derives from the noun *der Mann* (meaning a masculine person and reflecting the patriarchal ideology underlying social norms) and is used to denote cultural and public consensus about 'doing the right thing'. Discussing emotions, Ms M said: 'Except in the event of death where one is in mourning, I really can't say that I had ever been unhappy.' The lack of emotion, which had stabilized her life and acted as a shield against pain, protected Ms M in later life from the fear of death. A defensive process had already begun in that she would not let anything unusual, new, or strange get close to her. Although she had had a lot of dealings with young people, it is clear from her statements that she rejected them and their new and different ideas. She avoided contact with young people; 'No, I am at my best when I am around people of my own age group. I always have the feeling that young people lead entirely different kinds of lives . . . I understand my children's generation, but much younger people and their lifestyles are alien to me.' This could be interpreted as a strategy for maintaining her sense of equilibrium in later life.

Third case: Ms R

Background

Ms R was born in 1928 on the island of Sumatra, the child of a doctor and nurse who had immigrated to Indonesia two years before. She had one brother and lived there until 1940. In May of that year, the Germans marched into Holland and, as a Dutch colony, the inhabitants of Indonesia felt the effects of the war as well. Initially, Germans and Austrians were kept under surveillance by the Indonesians, then detained unless they could afford to leave the country. Encouraged by her father, who was forced to remain in Indonesia and lost his life in 1942, Ms R's mother made her way with both children to Vienna, where they began a new life. Secondary school, school-leaving exams, fashion school and apprenticeship exams were some of the key events in Ms R's early life. Because of an eye disease she was unable to practise her acquired profession, so she took a job in an office where she could put her knowledge of Dutch to use. Five years later she moved to a petroleum company, where she met her future husband. They married and had two children. After a few years, she began to work part time in a gallery and then obtained a job in the civil service, where she remained until her retirement. She then began to study sociology and in the process initiated a project, which is now established, for exchange between generations. The interview took place in the researcher's apartment, as this was convenient for Ms R. She seemed to be an open and active woman, who, judging by her appearance, had a pleasant lust for life.

Analysis and interpretation

Wonderful memories of her childhood came to an end with the return to Vienna, which took place under difficult conditions. Through the loss of her father, her mother became the most important reference person, whose strengths and weaknesses she was fully aware of. 'My mother was a very dominant person and it was a struggle; on the one hand, she could be very understanding, but then there were times when she found it difficult even to meet me halfway.' It was taken for granted, given the family's social background, that the sons would be supported through a university education. Ms R describes the obvious favour shown to the male members of the family thus: 'My brother studied anthropology. He could have studied the strangest thing, but that parental support would nonetheless have been a foregone conclusion.' Girls, on the other hand, were expected to learn a useful trade, rather than pursue an academic career. 'Oh yes, that was definitely assumed. Even though it was rarely mentioned, a girl was also expected to marry.' In the interval between leaving school and getting married, girls were expected to be in employment. 'My mother told me: "You should do something, that's quite clear"'. Ms R was also keen to work, partly because she wished to have financial independence: 'I was not a spoiled little rich girl who waited for a free ride. It was definitely not like that. In any case I wanted this for myself.'

Ms R's mother remained her role image throughout adulthood: 'Yes, she was a tremendous role model for me, what with her self-discipline – one who took her life in her own hands – she was just brought up that way. And I'm like that too.' Another role image mentioned by Ms R was that of Mother Theresa, simultaneously Madonna, saint and mother, although she was seen as; 'so high up, that I neither could nor would ever try to aspire to [her level]'. In seeing this image as unattainable, Ms R differentiated between the ideal and the practical aspects of life. Yet it was important to her to have children in order to achieve the mother role. 'Yes, I can say the desire to have children was very strong. If I couldn't have children myself, I wanted to adopt. I didn't want to let this opportunity slip by me.'

After the wedding, children and family demanded Ms R's full attention for a time. However, she became aware that childrearing no longer provided her with feelings of approval and fulfilment and that matrimony offered her no challenges.

> I didn't want to stay home, especially in view of the fact that my husband was like a bachelor with dependants and not in that sense a family man, as one would have liked to imagine it, and I said to myself, no, I'm not going to become one of those women who sits around in a coffee house all day and plays bridge.

After the 'family bubble', as she describes the period of total concentration on the children and family, had burst, she experienced a crisis. Adjustment to bourgeois patterns was not acceptable to her, so she searched for and found a new role: she wanted to have a career again.

Employment after leaving school was meant to be a 'bridge' leading to marriage, one's primary role in life, but when her family did not provide the fulfilment she had been led to expect by society, Ms R sought to meet her needs through a new career. 'I want to do something that I enjoy doing, that gives me a sense of acknowledgement.' Ms R did two things. First, she trusted her own feelings of dissatisfaction with her roles. Second, she dispensed with beliefs such as the one that 'never-ending happiness' is to be found in women's roles. It is likely that the effect of the women's liberation movement encouraged her aspirations. Consequently, she abandoned her role of being the centre of a happy family; her entry into public life marked a break with societal convention in that she placed her own wishes above those of her husband.

With the help of an older gentleman she found an interesting part time position in a gallery. Joining the workforce again was a significant step in that

> I didn't receive any support at all from my husband, he told me, 'Yes, go ahead and do it' but (typical macho) 'I don't have anything against it, as

long as the family doesn't suffer'. Hearing this, my ambition grew stronger and I thought to myself, I'll show you, and then I became confident – that was the first step to my self-autonomy.

Her husband found no reason to modify his patriarchal views. Ms R's struggle reflects social changes which led to a new societal role image: that of the 'super woman'. 'I don't know how, but it worked. Back then we had a dog . . . the children were in secondary school and I had to be at the gallery from 10 to 2 o'clock . . . how I did it I don't know, for three months it was really tough.' Ms R had responsibility for the household, the children and her own career but, unlike Ms U who worked to be needed, or Ms M who had to work for subsistence, Ms R wanted a career for self-development. She surmounted all the difficulties of combining a career and family and fulfilled her wishes and desires.

Retirement was no shock to her. Consciously, because it was of prime importance to her to do what she was interested in, she said to herself, 'there must be more to life than this' and began to study sociology. Ms R's process of ageing is noteworthy because her search for a re-evaluation of roles is removed from the 'do the right thing' mentality and leads her closer to her self, her interests, and her desires, which are all steps towards authenticity.

Ms R portrays her life story as one based on phases, in which the break with her idyllic childhood dreams plays an important part. That is the point from which she describes the establishment of a development process and thereby the ageing process (and older age itself), not as deterioration, but rather as a process of maturation and emancipation. Her understanding of this process is that established role images may be critically observed according to the meaning they have in one's own life, how they can be used for one's own purposes and whether one should reject or modify them. 'I was confronted with tasks that had to be accomplished. And there was no other possibility. I had two options, either to take control of my life and develop further, or become ill. I chose the first option.' She bases her conception of positive health on 'coming to terms' with herself: 'The doctor certainly can help a person, but the "will to live" that helps you to be healthy comes from inside oneself.' She doesn't put the responsibility for her own life on others, even though she does need to feel acknowledged by them. She is her own authority and she trusts mainly in herself. For her, getting older means the need to search for new possibilities. Will this be what 'to do the right thing' means in future?

At the end of the twentieth century a woman in her 60s expects to live about two decades more and has to face the task of giving meaning to this part of her life. In the future, the societal attitude concerning the participation of older people is likely to be more open-minded. Age boundaries in certain domains, for example in higher education, have largely lost their significance. Other roles besides that of the good grandmother or doing charitable work are open to older women. For example, Ms R at the age of 60 wished to develop her capabilities by attending university. Ageing liberated her from some of the burdens of women's roles. Unlike women born earlier, she encountered a social climate in which there was greater freedom and awareness of gender, so that individuals could seek 'new' ways according to their wishes.

Ms R embodies the image of the wise and supportive older woman who seeks contact with young people and, as a direct result of her own struggle for autonomy, wishes to communicate to others – but without dominating them – her wisdom and lust for life.

Summary and discussion

The first two cases represent patterns that conform to society's gender norms, although Ms M struggled hard to find her position in society because of her identification with her father and dislike of conventional feminine roles. There is some evidence in the women's histories to support Gutmann's (1987) thesis that women become more confident and assertive as they age, although Ms U remained conformist throughout her life. It seems that the women did not seek to defy convention in order to achieve authenticity but rather that they learnt to come to terms with their lives, finding an acceptable arrangement in earlier stages of the life course as well as in later life. Roles were reorganized in the time after retirement, although not necessarily by rebelling against society.

The difference between generations is shown in the case of Ms R, who, encouraged by changed social attitudes towards women and aware of her own ageing, broke away from society's traditional role images and sought a new lifestyle in her 40s. Her reactions to social role images were not completely different from those of the two other women; however, she took delight in the things she decided to do, following a course of action not because she was told to 'do the right thing' but because she wanted to 'do the right thing for herself'. The roles themselves did not change, as Ms R also acted in later life as a grandmother and wise older woman, but she performed the roles in a different way. As society became more liberal from the 1970s, social patterns were critically examined and new ways of fulfilling social roles developed in which autonomy and self-esteem were more important; this started a process of redefinition and change in the quality of gender roles.

In documenting women's images and how these change through historical time, we find clear correspondences between these images and women's social roles. The prevalence of the images is an indication of the importance to society of the fulfilment of women's roles. In performing their roles and in perpetuating the associated images, women serve as role models for the next generation, passing on the social prescriptions (MacPherson 1990) and thereby contributing to the structure of society.

The typical female role images are mainly found in the social and family domain, where the work performed by women is seen by society as being on a voluntary basis (Oakley 1974; MacDonald and Rich 1984), rewarded by the family in the form of praise or gifts. Most of the roles and functions found in the three case histories seem to be as applicable to older women as to younger:

- The 'good mother' or the 'good grandmother' is wholly involved in this role, undertaking all the social duties of the care and education of the children.
- The 'good daughter' takes over further social duties, such as caring for the sick and for frail older people (especially parents or parents-in-law), as purely a private responsibility. This role can also persist into older age, being expanded to include the care of siblings and friends.
- The 'good wife' is responsible for managing family life and in later years for the care of her husband.
- For older women especially, the 'wise older woman' and voluntary work outside the family provides an opportunity to give support and social assistance to others.
- Finally, the image of the 'hard worker' is important in the working world of the generation of Ms M and Ms U. Where employment is not an essential part of identity, the loss of this role can mean merely a relief from duties. However, where the psychological benefits of a job are important, for example in providing stability and confirmation of being needed, these must be replaced in order to avoid depression (Gallie and Vogler 1990).

These unpaid roles performed by women are fundamental to the maintenance of the existing social system in the West (Gee and Kimball 1987); they constitute an enormous amount of work which is largely invisible, reflecting the lack of recognition of women's contributions to society (Bassein 1993).

How the gender role images which influenced the lives of older women will be interpreted and changed by the next generation of women is becoming an increasingly important issue. What does ageing mean for women aged 30, 40, or 50 at the end of the twentieth century? And how do the needs of society and the demands of individual men confront women at different stages in the life course? A comparison of the expectations and demands made by society on women through their life course (Allatt et al. 1987) and how these are changing in a social and political context which has incorporated some elements of feminism (Mulqueen 1992) is important for understanding how ageing and gender are connected.

5

Gendered Work, Gendered Retirement

Miriam Bernard, Catherine Itzin, Chris Phillipson and Julie Skucha

In this chapter, we explore some of the ways in which gendered processes in the workplace influence the position of women in later life. In particular, it is our contention that the transition through to retirement reflects the working out of different forms of gender differentiation, with the influence of workplace structures and work experiences being of central importance in this process. Research has shown that these structures and experiences are undoubtedly decisive in terms of the reproduction of financial inequalities in retirement (Arber and Ginn 1991a; Henretta 1994), but they are also likely to influence wider issues concerning the marginalization of older women and their ability to take control of their lives (Bernard and Meade 1993).

It is this broader linkage which is the central concern of this chapter. We pursue this theme first through a brief review of the literature examining gender and the social construction of work and retirement. Second, drawing on findings from two research studies, we explore some of the connections between age, gender and employment by examining attitudes towards, and the experiences of, mature and older women workers in various settings. Finally, the chapter concludes with a review of policy issues and a research agenda for future studies.

Gender and the social construction of retirement

In the 1990s, the relationship between work and retirement is undergoing rapid change. Macro economic policies are consolidating the institutionalization of retirement, at the same time as cultural changes are loosening commitments to paid work amongst certain groups in industrial societies. The expected pattern for men of previous generations – long work, short retirement – is being dissolved (Schuller 1989), while the transition into retirement has come to be organized on a more flexible basis, with a range of pathways (such as part time working, unemployment, disability, redundancy) which people follow before they either describe themselves or are defined within the social security system as 'wholly retired' (Kohli *et al.* 1991; Atchley 1993; Phillipson 1994). Yet despite general agreement about the increasing diversity of pathways into retirement, there is less understanding or agreement about the potential role of key variables such as social class or gender in this process (Kohli and Rein 1991).

The role of gender seems especially important, for three main reasons. First, the types of paid work carried out by women may have considerable implications for the transition into retirement and their experience of later life (Martin and Roberts 1984; Itzin and Phillipson 1993). The British labour market is characterized by a number of gender-based inequalities. For example, the majority of women who are employed are located in low-status, low-paid, sex-segregated work which offers little opportunity to progress or prosper (Martin and Roberts 1984; Abdela 1991). The typecasting of women into subordinate roles at work is often age-related (Tyler and Abbott 1994), whilst various researchers also point to the clustering of women in jobs with limited or non-existent pensions (Stone and Minkler 1984; Davies and Ward 1992; Ginn and Arber 1993; Henretta 1994). Moreover, the growth of part time employment is one of the most important aspects of the recent work history of women in Britain (Elias and Gregory 1994). Women comprised 86 per cent of the part time workforce in the late 1980s and, in contrast with their European counterparts, British women were much more likely to be engaged in part time rather than full time employment during the later phases of their working lives (Department of Employment 1991).

Second, Szinovacz (1991) notes that the discontinuous nature of women's work histories means that many women come to regard their mid-life as a special challenge and opportunity, and may view the later phase of their work career in a different way from men. They are also less likely than men to have achieved their career goals at the time their spouses wish to retire, or when employers' retirement incentives encourage their husband's retirement.

Third, gender differences in adjustment to retirement have been reported by a number of researchers. Szinovacz (1982) provided one of the first reviews of this issue. Jacobson's (1974) British study in the early 1970s found that women with a strong social attachment to the workplace were less willing to retire than those without, and were less likely than men to be positively orientated to retirement. In the USA, Streib and Schneider (1971) found women to be more apprehensive than men about the effects of retirement and Atchley (1976) found women taking longer than men to adapt to the retirement transition, findings confirmed in Fox's (1976) research on the adaptation of women workers to retirement. The dynamics of the retirement decision are different for women and men because of their dissimilar financial positions; Atchley (1982) suggests that whereas men who work beyond state pension age do so mainly because of enjoyment of their work, women who delay retirement are more likely to do so because of a low pension entitlement.

Gender, work and organizational culture

An additional influence on women's retirement, running through all the above factors, is that of workplace structures and women's experiences of work itself. Here, there are two contrasting views which seem to be emerging in terms of the relative positions of men and women as they move through the life course. On the one hand, there is what may loosely be described as a 'convergence model' whereby younger cohorts of women are seen to be experiencing the kind of life course segmentation – with the division between education, work and retirement – which has long been characteristic of men. Such a view also emphasizes the growth of flexible patterns of work, together with an increase in part time working, both of which are seen to be areas of growth for men and women in the middle and older age groups (Laczko and Phillipson 1991).

The alternative perspective, although accepting the significance of the above changes, would note that they take place within a social structure which produces and maintains gender differences (Itzin and Newman 1995). According to this perspective, we need to understand the way in which changes to work and retirement reflect gendered arrangements which actively create and maintain differences between individual women and men throughout the life course.

One issue here concerns the impact on women of work organization and culture. Research has demonstrated the extent to which sexual discrimination is embedded within the cultures of organizations (Abdela 1984; Reskin and Padavic 1994). There have been studies on male domination in a variety of forms, relating to ownership and control, status and authority and cultural values (Morgan, G. 1986; Hearn *et al.* 1989; Crompton and Sanderson 1990). Mills (1989: 33) sees gender 'permeating not only extra-organizational rules, but each and every area of rule bound behaviour' in organizations, and he cites research showing how women may be denied access to organizational networks (Simpson *et al.* 1987); that access to informal knowledge and networks depends on participation in male-oriented social activities (Crompton and Jones 1984); that men rather than women benefit from the advice of mentors in the workplace (Noe 1988), and that the motivating language of the organization may be communicated in terms of male-oriented metaphors (Riley 1983). In addition, it is clear that the occupational profiles of women do not fit neatly with organizational expectations (Martin and Roberts 1984; Cunnison 1987; Lemmer 1991), and that attempts to improve the position of women within organizations through equal opportunities policies meets with resistance from men (Cockburn 1991). Recent research has conceptualized the various forms of male domination within organizations in terms of a 'gender culture' and analysed the effect of gendered power relations on organizational culture, structure and practices (Itzin and Newman 1995).

Women of all ages are affected by sex discrimination in employment and older people, both male and female, are affected by age discrimination. Increasingly, however, there has been a growing interest in the extent to which a form of 'gendered ageism' operates against women in particular (Bernard and Meade, 1993; Itzin and Phillipson 1993, 1995; Tyler and Abbott 1994). This has manifested itself primarily in studies of the employment situation of older women (Harrop 1990; Arber and Ginn 1991a; Bernard and Meade, 1993). There is also increasing evidence that age combines with gender to disadvantage women within organizations at all ages (Itzin 1986; Itzin and Phillipson 1995). This pattern of discrimination is likely to be decisive in shaping a range of experiences affecting women in work and retirement.

In line with this, we move now to consider the connection between gendered work and gendered retirement – and the transition between the two. Following Reskin and Padavic (1994), we call the process of gender differentiation 'gendering' and speak of activities that organizations have attached to one or other sex as 'gendered'. Accordingly, 'these terms signify outcomes that are socially constructed and give males advantages over females. They describe the production of assumptions about gender as well as the institutions that are shaped by those assumptions' (Reskin and Padavic 1994: 6). In order to explore these issues further, we draw on findings from two recent research studies which both look at the connections between age, gender and employment and examine attitudes towards, and the experiences of, mature and older women workers in various settings.

Researching the connections between age, gender and employment

In this section we briefly discuss the design and methods employed in the two research studies. The first, commissioned by the Metropolitan Authorities Recruitment Agency (referred to hereafter as the METRA study), was a large scale national study examining the position of mature and older male and female workers in the context of local government (Itzin and Phillipson 1993). By contrast, our second study was a small scale exploratory investigation, supported by the Pre-Retirement Association of Great Britain and Northern Ireland (referred to hereafter as the PRA study). It examined some of the ways in which the transition into later life of mature and older women part time workers might be assisted through formal preparation programmes (Skucha et al. in press).

The METRA study had three major phases. The first phase involved a postal survey to all local authorities in England and Wales and was carried out in the spring of 1992. Of 449 authorities, 221 completed the questionnaire, a response rate of 49 per cent. The second phase involved case study fieldwork in a representative sample of 11 local authorities. Each case study looked at the corporate policies and practices of the authority and then focused on the particular situations within different service departments. Tape recorded in-depth interviews were held with managers, and group interviews were conducted with older employees in senior management, in administrative and clerical work, and in manual work. Group interviews were also carried out with women aged 35–50 in middle management. Overall, around 350 people were interviewed in one form or another in the case studies. The third phase involved a self-completion questionnaire sent to 476 senior managers in eight of the 11 service departments selected for the case study research. Three hundred and three questionnaires were completed giving a response rate of 64 per cent.

The PRA study, being smaller in scope and time, was divided into two main phases of data collection. The first comprised a series of tape recorded guided interviews with an opportunity sample of 31 women, aged between 45 and 62, drawn from six public and private sector organizations in the West Midlands. The interviews were undertaken in March 1993 at the women's places of work, and comprised nine individual and six group interviews. Information from these interviews was then used to develop a postal questionnaire for the second phase of the research. Two organizations from phase one participated (a council and a cleaning firm), together with an additional borough council. In May 1993, questionnaires were distributed to 225 female employees (75 in each organization) of which 62 questionnaires were returned. This low response rate (28 per cent) appears to be connected with the considerable reorganization and restructuring of the workforces amongst the surveyed organizations, and with the way in which the distribution and return of some questionnaires was mediated via management personnel – issues which are discussed more fully elsewhere (Skucha et al. in press).

Both the METRA study and the PRA study yielded a great deal of data. The findings presented here are, of necessity, selective and concentrate largely on the qualitative elements. We now draw on these findings to discuss three broad areas: first, management views of the impact of gender and age on employment; second, women's own experiences inside organizations and the role of employment in their lives; and third, the links between women's working lives and their lives in retirement.

The management view

The connection of gender and age was very clearly revealed when line managers in the METRA study, 68 per cent of whom were male and 32 per cent were female (n=303), were asked whether they regarded specific kinds of jobs as more or less suitable to older workers. Most of the answers reflected sex-segregated work. Older women were regarded as more suitable for clerical, caring, cleaning and catering work, and as less suitable than men for chief executive and senior management jobs or for heavy manual work as porters, caretakers, or road workers. Predictably, the majority of women in both the public and the private sectors in this study and all women in the PRA study were employed in positions that were regarded as suitable for them. What is also disturbing is that some women had internalized these beliefs and expectations about gender and age-appropriate work. A number of the part time workers in the PRA study regarded 'women's work', which they described as low status and low paid, as inferior compared with that of men. Men, they contended, would not accept the kind of jobs they did. As one clerical worker put it: 'Women are prepared to take any work they can do if they need the money. Men tend to be too choosy'. They had great difficulty in envisaging themselves as on a par with men, and placed themselves in the middle of 'a hierarchy of valuable workers' – below men, but above young people. Paradoxically, although they argued that women would go to greater lengths than men to obtain employment, none of them would go so far as to identify paid work as more important to women than men regardless of earnings differentials.

One (male) manager in the METRA study described the over representation of women in lower grades in his authority as a 'traditional ladies' horror story of 60 per cent plus of the women in clerical jobs with little prospect of progression'. One manager observed that it tended to be older women who were located in administrative and clerical posts, while another commented that the 'council has a hard core in administration, often long-serving "middle-aged" women who are seen as set in their ways'. When another authority had set up a development programme for staff on scales one to four, over 90 per cent of these were women over 40. 'It's clear that something is operating to keep women in lower grades and it's both age and gender issues that affect where and when women plateau in an organization', said one female head of personnel.

The glass ceiling of age

The notion of where and when women 'plateau' in an organization, and the promotion barriers which they experience along the way, is encapsulated in the concept of the 'glass ceiling of age'. An important finding from the METRA study was that, in general terms, women were perceived as being 'older earlier' than men and it was mainly men rather than women who thought this to be the case. Women generally come up against a barrier to further promotion at an earlier age than men. As the director of personnel in one authority put it: 'Women hit their peak younger than men' and 'Women get where they are going by the age of 35'. This finding was supported in the survey of line managers, a few of whom categorized women as 'older workers' from the age of 30. They also tended to view women in their 40s, rather more than men at this age, as being 'older workers'. However, managers' gender bias in perception of age was most pronounced in regard to women in their 50s. These perceptions and expectations often appear to be internalized by women themselves. Indeed, many of the respondents in the PRA study regarded 30 or 35 as the age at which women entered the category of 'older worker'.

Broken careers and the golden decade

In addition to the discriminatory potential inherent in the perception of women as ageing earlier and being older at a younger age than men, the majority of women will at some time in their reproductive life bear and rear children, many taking a break from employment for part of their childrearing years. A service director in an authority committed to age equality described a woman assistant director who 'took maternity leave one year after appointment' and commented that 'this wasn't well received'. A personnel officer said 'all the women now come back after their statutory maternity entitlement', and were wary of taking longer career breaks. Another service director said,

> career breaks can adversely affect women depending on how long they decide to stay out of work. If they stay out for a number of years, it may be difficult for them to get back in. Women's careers are fragmented and do not follow the straighter path of men's.

The service director of one authority described the career break as 'a handicap for women', while another said he 'would like to think the career break wasn't a barrier, but it is'.

Alongside this, women also have to confront the notion of a 'golden decade'; 'there is now a culture that our top managers come in at around 40 and we tend to appoint people in their golden decade [i.e. 30/35–40/45]', said the head of personnel in an authority with a high-profile commitment to countering age discrimination in employment. 'Chief executives are appointed at 45-ish', said one manager, 'and most chief officers by 40'. He added: 'Members just aren't prepared to contemplate anyone over the age of 40.' A chief personnel officer put it even more bluntly, adding that: 'The cut-off point for women's career progression is 10 years younger than for men.' It seems, therefore, that age restrictions combine with the handicapping effects of career breaks to exert considerable constraints on women's promotion opportunities. The price often paid by women who do achieve senior positions was vividly illustrated by a male personnel officer: 'If they are going to play the male game, and at the moment they have no choice, women have to put off having children until they are 30.' Another manager described women as, 'five to ten years late in their careers if they have taken a break, perhaps having spent their golden decade at home with children and ready for a golden decade at work some ten years later than men'. A female chief officer with two children was only able to return to work by using nannies, an option not available to most women.

A female head of personnel said she and the other two 'women at the top' all had caring commitments, but had not taken a break from work in spite of the authority's positive and encouraging policy on career breaks. They recognized that in practice a break in career was a liability: 'The golden decade can't apply to women if they have had a break.'

These findings create the strong impression that women's employment and career development opportunities are often determined by structural and situational factors which are not of their own making, and which may not meet their own needs and preferences. Women's careers are blocked in ways that men's are not and they feel that, unless they are prepared to 'play the male game', they will continue to suffer discrimination by managers. This highlights the conflict which still exists between official personnel policy on equal opportunities, and the harsh reality of the workplace for many women.

The experience of women

In this section we consider further the experiences of women in the differing organizations for which they worked, and highlight the importance of employment to women despite its manifest difficulties and constraints. The METRA case study data brought out a number of important issues about the experience of women inside organizations. 'Whatever age they are, women's age is held against them. They are never the right age, they are either too young or too old', said one woman in a statement which seems to epitomize the attitude of management, as revealed by our interviews. As we have observed previously, the effects of this 'gendered ageism' adversely influence women's conditions of work and career opportunities.

Women provided many examples of how ageing is gendered. In particular, it is viewed negatively for women in a way that does not occur for men: 'Men don't take you seriously as you get older', suggested one woman. 'They see you as you were 10 years ago. I'm still asked to do routine tasks, even though I have obtained qualifications and am in a much more senior post.' 'I went to an interview', said another, 'and it was quite evident that they wanted a young attractive woman.' From another authority, a woman said: 'Men don't want women at the top. They pay lip service to equal opportunities, but they think if you are a woman you are only good for pushing pens and making tea.' In one authority the women reported that the male assistant director 'won't employ women of child-bearing years'. One woman had been asked when she applied for a post at the age of 24 whether she was in a steady relationship and planning to have children. If only women are asked such questions, this is sex discrimination and unlawful under the 1975 legislation.

Gendered ageism also has profoundly negative effects on women's own attitudes, beliefs and behaviour. 'Women tend to look at their disadvantages rather than what they have to offer', was how one woman put it, while another said, 'You don't want to look like you are past your sell-by-date.' In the words of a third woman:

> Women are made to feel they have not done things at the right age. Not married at 30? No children at 40? These pressures affect women's self-image. Women feel obliged to dye their hair. Age is a visible issue, others define you negatively if you look older, women much more so and much earlier than men. Women can overcome some of the disadvantages of age-stereotyping at work by looking younger as long as they can.

For the women in the PRA study, the influences of age and gender were also apparent. The difficulties attendant on taking employment breaks to have and rear children are but one example of this. In the interviews, the women discussed these experiences in detail, describing the problems of their skills becoming outmoded; the prohibitive costs of retraining – especially with child care expenses to cover; and the loss of confidence in their dealings with 'the outside world' after such breaks. For them, whether to work part time or full time was rarely a matter of choice; instead, it represented the most convenient way of coping with the combination of their domestic and caring responsibilities and their need to earn money. Part time working and breaks in employment undoubtedly have consequences both for women's chances of occupational success and for their pension income when they retire.

Working lives and retirement lives

The way in which gendered processes at work create and sustain inequalities as women move into retirement is a key concern of this chapter. Although retirement was not a specific focus of the METRA study, there was evidence from the case study data that early retirement was being used as a 'management tool' in several authorities. The reasons given for offering early retirement included 'poor performance', 'people who won't change', and physical decline. However, the most common reason given was reorganization and restructuring, which closely reflects the reasons why certain organizations were reluctant to take part in the PRA study. Early retirement can have considerable impact on individuals: the short term attraction of escaping from the stresses and uncertainties of later working life might well be appealing, but early retirement may also lead to an increased risk of poverty in old age (Laczko 1990). For many women in the METRA study, who had re-entered the labour market after childrearing, or who had worked part time in manual jobs, the prospect of a limited pension made early retirement a poor option.

The respondents in the PRA study saw early exit from the labour market as a desirable option if, and only if, financial circumstances were sufficiently good. 'If it's choice, then that's fine. But, I don't think that anybody should feel there's a gentle boot under them to push them because they've reached a certain age', commented one interviewee. It was also regarded as a more attractive option if the woman had a partner who was also retired, so that they had each other's company. In the absence of either or both of these conditions, most respondents preferred to work on until statutory pension age. The timing of retirement was generally viewed by these women to be dependent upon circumstances at the time, and therefore not a decision they could predict.

Retirement, and women's attitudes towards it, formed a major focus of the PRA study. Respondents were asked to describe their reaction to the word 'retirement', and to compare their expected later life with that of men of the same age. Where women expressed positive reactions, these focused on the time and freedom to be enjoyed. Increased autonomy and reduced pressure were expected to combine to create a relaxed lifestyle which, many stressed, would nonetheless be an active period of life. They hoped for the renewal of relationships with their partners, a time in which they would be free of parental responsibilities and able to travel and socialize together. By contrast, negative reactions emphasized isolation, the lack of structure formerly provided by employment, and the undesirable aspects of ageing. Fear and dread were recurrent themes, with retirement conjuring up images of 'old ladies sitting around in chairs, drinking tea. Terrifying thought', wrote one office manager. 'I think of boredom. Dreading it!' replied an assistant cook.

The women's views on gender differences in adjustment to, and enjoyment of, retirement were also illustrative of the meaning retirement held for them. Many thought that women were able to make the adjustment more easily for two reasons. These were, first, that work had played a less central role in their life, and second, that women were used to making the necessary adjustments to living without paid employment. Significantly, however, being retired was seen as easier for men, since they were free to concentrate on their leisure; women, on the other hand, were expected to continue with their responsibility for motivating and organizing life for themselves and their household (see Mason 1987, for similar findings). 'It is different. I think it's more of a holiday for a man than a woman because a woman still carries the burden of a home', and 'A woman is more motivated to doing things . . . but men never seem to motivate themselves', were two illustrative comments.

A predominant attitude was that women do not actually retire in the sense of stopping work, because women continue with their domestic responsibilities. This indicates the extent to which women's attitudes toward retirement have been shaped by traditional gender roles. Laczko and Phillipson's (1991) finding that the majority of non-employed older women would not describe them-selves as retired, even up to age 74, has two possible explanations. Either the women had not engaged in paid work prior to reaching the statutory pension age, or they felt that retirement, with its implications of leisure and freedom from obligation to perform (unpaid) work, did not describe the reality of their existence. Our findings support the latter explanation. Furthermore, there is a strong suggestion that the women rejected the applicability of the term 'retiree' to women as a group.

In summary, our findings show that both working lives and retirement are affected by age and gender considerations. Most of the women in the PRA study had experienced strictly gendered working lives and, whilst they were hoping for a less gendered retirement, they still expected their later lives to be predominantly organized according to traditional gender roles. In the light of this, we turn, in the concluding section of this chapter, to a consideration of policy and research issues.

Gendered work and retirement: Research and policy agendas

Both the studies discussed above led to a series of detailed recommendations concerning policy and research. The recommendations arising from the METRA study are oriented towards the development of an effective employment policy for mature and older workers of both sexes. By contrast, the PRA study was primarily concerned with how preretirement education could most effectively be delivered to mature and older women workers. However, both studies highlight a number of related policy issues. These concern first, the overriding need for equal opportunities in all aspects of employment, including recruitment, career development and at the stage of leaving work; second, the need for active development and maintenance of organizational cultures sensitive to the needs of mature women workers in particular, and older people in general (Itzin and Newman 1995); third, measures to prevent the widespread income poverty which currently exists amongst women in later life; and fourth, the need to improve access to training and continuing education, including preretirement education.

Underlying these recommendations are two core principles. First, all these suggestions call for a broad understanding and appreciation of the ways in which age and gender interact in constructing present organizational policies and practices, which affect both work and retirement. Second, if positive change is to come about, it is crucial that mature and older workers (both male and female) are treated first and foremost as human resources, rather than as expendable commodities within the workforce (Laczko and Phillipson 1991; Itzin and Phillipson 1993).

The policy issues outlined above have implications for applied research, particularly studies evaluating specific policy and practice measures. More broadly, we also need to recognize that the basis for research into the transition between work and retirement is changing rapidly, through a combination of developments in economic and social policy and transformations in individual attitudes and behaviour. Our understanding of these changes and inter-relationships is fragmented and imperfect and, for researchers, they present important challenges for further study. Three issues in particular may be identified.

First, the research we have discussed here concentrates on women in paid employment. In a British context, there is great scope for additional research on groups like mature and older part time women workers about whom we know comparatively little. The challenges of the retirement transition for professional women, and for dual earner couples are also little understood. Alongside this, some consideration is also merited of mature and older women who are outside the paid labour market, but whose successful adjustment to later life might also benefit from various forms of sensitive assistance such as is increasingly being offered through preretirement education.

Second, the conceptual and theoretical relationships between paid work and retirement need clarification. Both the METRA study and the PRA study have implicitly accepted the traditional definitions of these socially constructed divisions in the life course. This was a necessary prerequisite to the recognition of women's involvement in the labour market, but raises difficulties when paid work is not the central life interest, but only one of many important roles. Similarly, the concept of retirement as an event which primarily affects men has been absorbed into the consciousness of many women themselves, despite evidence from the (predominantly American) literature cited earlier which shows that it may be an equally difficult transition for women. This suggests that we need to challenge traditional conceptualizations for they have, to a great extent, conditioned the kinds of research carried out so far. In exploring the impact of age and gender over the latter phases of the life course, it may be more fruitful to move away from rigid distinctions between work and retirement, towards an alternative approach which gives greater priority to the interconnectedness of the spheres which make up our lives. This opens up the possibility of developing new theoretical constructions rather than continuing to rely on previous models and theories (Bernard and Meade 1993; Itzin and Newman 1995).

Third, an explicit examination of the intersection between gendered work and gendered retirement is lacking. Gendered work, which includes the sexual division of labour, the devaluation of women's work and the construction of gendered jobs in the workplace, has been subject to scrutiny by writers and researchers over the years. By contrast, issues concerning gender and ageing have received only scant attention in the British literature until recently (Arber and Ginn 1991a; Bernard and Meade 1993). What is clear from the research so far is that women's financial circumstances in retirement are largely determined by their employment patterns (Ginn and Arber 1993, 1994a, 1994b). The double jeopardy of age and gender discrimination highlighted in both the METRA and PRA studies means that older women, with their characteristically interrupted employment careers and low earnings, will have very limited potential to enjoy what are now being increasingly promoted as the benefits of retirement. The agenda should now move beyond the reproduction of financial inequalities and begin to investigate systematically the ways in which gendered work affects other aspects of life in retirement. This would include examination of hitherto little explored areas such as housing and accommodation as well as leisure and education. It would also need to take us beyond description of what the links might be, to ask more pertinently, how and why this should be so.

Overall, what is important to establish is that work and retirement, and the transition between the two, is undergoing radical alteration as we move towards the twenty-first century. Gender and age considerations are becoming more important, yet it is still difficult for us to grasp the scale of these changes and their impact on individual attitudes and behaviour. The challenge for researchers is an exciting one: to document new patterns of work and retirement, whilst at the same time contributing to the emerging debates about how we might theorize the wider relationships between age and gender in the future.

6

CHOICE AND CONSTRAINT IN THE RETIREMENT OF OLDER MARRIED WOMEN

Sara Arber and Jay Ginn

The social norm of the male breadwinner with a wife engaged in homemaking is weaker now than earlier this century. Nevertheless, in spite of the widespread acceptance of the principle of equal opportunities and increasing employment of married women, it is still rare for wives to be main or equal breadwinners (Arber and Ginn 1995a) and the situation where a man stays at home while his wife goes out to work is still regarded as strange and undesirable by many. Such a reversal of 'traditional' gender roles may be seen as challenging husbands' economic dominance, a longstanding source of patriarchal power and masculine identity, as well as a justification for minimal involvement in domestic work.

A key issue is the extent to which such considerations apply to couples around pensionable age and influence the timing of the retirement of each spouse. Are wives likely to remain in the labour market when their husbands have already retired?

Research on younger couples has shown that the wives of unemployed men are less likely to be employed than other married women (McKee 1987; Morris 1989, 1990). Shifts in the domestic division of labour (especially childcare), in families where wives are in paid employment and their husbands are not, are culturally unacceptable and strongly resisted. Other factors besides the social norm of the male breadwinner may contribute to the concentration of non-employment in couples. First, social security rules based on the assumption of wives' financial dependence are likely to have a disincentive effect on women's employment where their partners are unemployed; means testing of joint income ensures that wives' earnings would only increase the couple's income if her earnings were high enough to compensate for loss of Income Support and Housing Benefit (Morris 1990). Second, wives' and husbands' employment tends to be equally affected by labour market conditions in specific geographical areas (Gallie *et al.* 1994). Third, recent research suggests similarity in the characteristics of marital partners: 'men who tend to experience unemployment (low skilled, unqualified, experience of many different jobs) are more likely . . . to marry women who have a low level of attachment to the labour market' (Davies *et al.* 1992).

Thus British research on couples where the husband is unemployed provides reasons to expect that older married women would leave the labour market either before or at the same time as their husband. It is important to examine couples' patterns of retirement timing: to what extent do partners time their exit so as to conform to traditional gender norms, avoiding a reversal of roles? This chapter will first contrast the meaning of retirement for women and men, and second, consider to what extent women's retirement is constrained by their husband's employment status.

Men's and women's retirement

Men's retirement and the extent to which men have left the labour market prior to state pension age has been a major focus of research attention in Britain (e.g. Laczko and Phillipson 1991) and in Europe (Kohli *et al.* 1991). However, there has been little British attention devoted to women's retirement and exit from the labour force, or to whether the retirement timing of wives is related to that of their husbands. This lack of interest is surprising, given the trends towards increased employment participation of women. American literature has long recognized that women's retirement cannot be treated as the same as men's, nor dismissed as unimportant on the grounds that women can return to the alternative role of housewife following retirement (Szinovacz 1982; 1987; Szinovacz *et al.* 1992).

Women's employment in Britain, although typically interrupted by a period of childbearing, is increasingly followed by a return to employment, often part time (Martin and Roberts 1984), with a peak rate of employment of over 70 per cent among women in their late 40s (discussed later). Thus women commonly have some financial independence during their working life. However, this independence is lost on retirement if they lack entitlements to state and occupational or personal pensions; this is the case for many women, due to their interrupted and part time employment patterns as well as to the way pension schemes are designed (Ginn and Arber 1991, 1993; Davies and Ward 1992). The period after intensive childrearing, usually from age 45, is one in which women can potentially improve their pension position (Ginn and Arber 1994a). Therefore, if women are constrained to leave the labour market early, for example because of their husband's retirement, they not only reduce their current income but also jeopardize their financial independence and well-being in later life through reducing the years in which they can build up entitlements to state and other pensions.

Men in most patriarchal societies tend to marry women who are younger than themselves, a tradition associated with the maintenance of a power differential within marriage. If women and men retired at the same age, this would clearly lead to husbands retiring before their wives, running counter to norms as to gender roles. In many countries, women's state pension age is lower than men's, so that despite the marital age differential, wives tend to leave work before their husbands. In Britain, the pension ages were set in 1940 at 60 for women and 65 for men (Thane 1978). Husbands are now on average two years older than their wives. Therefore, if each spouse retires at their state pension age and the wife is two years younger, she would retire three years earlier than her husband. A wife would have to be more than five years younger than her husband for retirement at state pension age to result in her working after her husband's retirement. Thus the current pension age differential reduces the chance of role reversal which could otherwise result from the marital age differential.

In practice, both women and men generally leave the labour market before state pension age, often due to ageist employer policies; there is evidence of age barriers limiting job opportunities for women over age 55 (Ginn and Arber, in press; and see Chapter 5 by Bernard *et al.*).

Theoretical approaches to women's retirement timing

American literature on women's retirement timing was originally located in a functionalist conception of the complementarity of gender roles, with women's financial dependence on their husband viewed as an acceptable arrangement. However, feminist theory, in which prescribed gender roles are seen as beneficial to patriarchy and/or capitalism but as oppressive to women, may provide a better framework. Like functionalist theory, feminist theory argues that the cultural norm of the husband retiring later than his wife or at the same time is supported by familial ideology as to the appropriate relative economic power of spouses; a wife continuing in paid employment after her husband's retirement challenges his status as chief economic provider. Such 'non-normative' retirement timing may also imply role reversal in terms of domestic labour, so that retired men with working wives may feel pressured to perform tasks generally undertaken by women. Unlike functionalist theory, feminist theory recognizes conflicts of interest within the family; a reversal of the gender roles associated with patriarchy is likely to be unwelcome to men (and possibly to their wives as well) and may therefore be resisted.

Alternatives to functionalist and patriarchal theories include ideas based on exchange theory and affinity theories (Henretta and O'Rand 1983). These two approaches suggest more symmetry in role relationships. Exchange theory is 'more flexible in its assumptions regarding the distribution of status and the negotiation of conjugal roles than the functional perspective' (p. 506). Affinity (or relational) theories suggest that gender symmetry is likely to develop where both partners are employed; 'to the degree that husbands and wives have similar roles, their behaviours are likely to be similar because of these similar roles' (p. 507). Both approaches imply symmetry and reciprocity: the characteristics of each spouse would be expected to have a similar effect on the retirement pattern of their partner, irrespective of gender.

Most American literature on retirement timing is framed in terms of partners' 'choice'; for example, Szinovacz (1989: 286) sees 'retirement timing of married couples as a decision outcome evolving from influence and negotiation processes between spouses'. However, Szinovacz does recognize limitations on choice, distinguishing between voluntary and non-voluntary retirement:

> retirement timing can be nonvoluntary as in the case of mandatory retirement or severe illness or disability of one or both spouses . . . nonvoluntary retirement of one spouse may require the other spouse to leave the labor force or to postpone retirement, regardless of his or her preferences (e.g., the spouse's illness demands extensive care giving).
>
> (Szinovacz 1989: 289)

Genuine choice in timing is therefore only possible where retirement is voluntary for both partners.

In Britain, couples' retirement timing is likely to be more constrained than in the US, since the majority of men and women who leave employment before the state pension age do so involuntarily, due to redundancy/dismissal, poor health or termination of a temporary job (Laczko and Phillipson 1991). In addition, many who take early retirement do so when their employer cuts back on staff, a situation which may allow very little choice. Those who retire at the state pension age generally leave employment at the mandatory retirement age for their job (Bone *et al.* 1992), again reflecting little choice in retirement timing. Throughout the European Union, there is a trend to early exit from the labour market (Drury 1993). The mode of exit and degree of choice is socially structured; whereas men in higher non-manual occupations tend to leave through 'early retirement' schemes, men in manual occupations are more likely to leave because of ill-health or redundancy (Arber 1989; Laczko and Phillipson 1991).

Thus the assumption in most of the US literature that retirement is voluntary, giving couples freedom to decide on how they time their exit in relation to each other, is less applicable in Britain; the majority of labour market exit is non-voluntary and its timing is therefore relatively constrained.

Gender differences in retirement timing

A range of mainly qualitative studies support the functionalist and patriarchal models of married women's retirement timing in relation to their husband.

Szinovacz (1989) graphically illustrates how some husbands in the US pressure their wives into 'joint' retirement, that is, retirement of both partners at about the same time; they are dissatisfied with the continued employment of their wives, resenting implied shifts in provider-role responsibilities. In some cases husbands make a unilateral decision that their wives should retire at the same time, while in others the pressure is more subtle and wives themselves say that they would prefer to retire at the same time to 'look after' their husband or enjoy leisure time together.

A small scale study of British women aged 50 to 69 (Mason 1987) suggested that there was considerable pressure on wives to retire at the same time as their husband. Husbands found it undesirable to be at home 'by themselves' while their wife went out to work and wives often also felt it was inappropriate.

Where retirement is 'joint', it is difficult to be certain of the relative influence of each partner on the retirement decision. Joint timing may result either from equally shared decision-making or from wives being persuaded to retire at the same time as their husband. However, the weight of evidence seems to point to the latter process. In the US, Shaw (1984) examined the retirement plans of middle-aged women, noting that some women said their husbands' retirement might influence their own retirement transitions. Similarly, the British Retirement and Retirement Plans Survey (Bone *et al.* 1992) reports that a small proportion of wives (under 10 per cent) said that their retirement was planned to coincide with their husbands' retirement, but no husbands reported a comparable influence on their retirement timing.

Some American research (Henretta and O'Rand 1983; O'Rand *et al.* 1992) has found symmetry in the determinants of retirement timing. For example, among couples where one spouse lacked private pension coverage, that partner tended to work longer; the greater the age gap between spouses, the higher the likelihood that the younger spouse would work longer; and the lower the wages of one spouse, the more likely that spouse would work longer. In all these patterns, the gender of the spouse had little effect. However, this research restricted attention to dual employed couples, defined as couples where the wife was in employment at age 55 (O'Rand *et al.* 1992). Couples with a more traditional employment pattern, in which the wife had left employment at some time prior to age 55, were excluded from consideration.

O'Rand *et al.*'s (1992) longitudinal study of couples where both partners were employed at age 55 found that 22 per cent had joint retirement (defined as leaving employment within 18 months of each other), 32 per cent were traditional, with the husband retiring after his wife, and in 31 per cent of couples, the wife retired after her husband. (The remaining 15 per cent of couples were both still in employment.) Joint retirement was associated with relative affluence, where the couples could afford to retire, and where the partners had been married for a long time and had rarely been married more than once. Wives who worked longer than their husbands tended to live in poorer households, suggesting they continued to work because the household was dependent on their earnings. They were more likely to have children under 21 in the household, to be married to men with health problems and to be closer in age to their husband. The traditional pattern was also associated with economic disadvantage and in this group some wives had left employment to provide care for other household members. Both these non-joint patterns were interpreted as reflecting constraint rather than choice in retirement timing.

Methods

This chapter first examines the gendered nature of retirement, focusing on how defining oneself as retired varies for older women and men. Second, we analyse the extent to which couples follow each of three patterns of final exit from paid employment: joint (or synchronous) retirement; the traditional sequence, in which the husband retires after his wife; and the non-traditional, where the wife retires later than her husband. Only 1 per cent of women aged 55–69 are cohabiting; we therefore include cohabiting couples with the married and refer to cohabiting women as wives.

The chapter uses data from the General Household Survey (OPCS 1992) and the Retirement and Retirement Plans Survey (Bone et al. 1992; ESRC Data Archive 1994a, 1994b). The General Household Survey interviews all adults aged 16 and over in a representative British sample of approximately 10,000 private households each year, with a response rate of about 82 per cent (OPCS 1992). The Retirement Survey interviewed a nationally representative sample of 55–69 year-old men and women, living in private households between November 1988 and January 1989: a total of 3542 respondents. In addition, over 600 partners outside this age range were interviewed. Respondents were asked for a full employment history and for the ages when they considered themselves to be retired and when they were last in paid employment.

The gendered nature of retirement

In line with the trend towards early exit from the labour market, the employment participation of both men and women in the early 1990s declines from age 50 onwards, well before the state pension age (Table 6.1). By age 60–64 only 39 per cent of men were in full time work, and under a quarter of women aged 55–59 worked full time, with a slightly larger proportion working part time. Thus, in the five years before state pension age (65 for men, 60 for women), only a minority of men (45 per cent) and half of women were in paid employment.

Although state pension age is not the key determinant of employment participation in mid-life, it does influence whether people consider themselves to be retired. Among men in their late 50s, only 7 per cent said they were

Table 6.1   Employment participation by age for women and men over 40

(a) Women

	Age							
	40–44 %	45–49 %	50–54 %	55–59 %	60–64 %	65–69 %	70–74 %	75+ %
Full time	38	40	32	23	7	1	–	–
Part time	35	35	34	29	15	6	3	1
Unemployed	4	3	3	3	–	–	–	–
Housewife	19	18	20	24	26	24	28	37
Other non-active (e.g. disabled)	4	4	8	11	1	1	1	2
Retired	–	–	2	10	51	68	68	60
N =	1728	1707	1402	1309	1258	1325	1139	1964

(b) Men

	Age							
	40–44 %	45–49 %	50–54 %	55–59 %	60–64 %	65–69 %	70–74 %	75+ %
Full time	85	85	78	64	39	5	1	–
Part time	2	2	3	4	6	8	5	1
Unemployed	7	6	7	10	6	–	–	–
Other non-active (e.g. disabled)	6	7	10	15	21	1	1	1
Retired	–	–	1	7	29	86	93	97
N =	1690	1581	1330	1295	1189	1122	895	1214

Source: General Household Survey, 1991–92 (authors' analysis). In these tables some of the column percentages do not add up to 100 per cent because of rounding.

retired compared with 25 per cent who were unemployed or not in the labour force for other reasons, such as disability. For men in their early 60s, these proportions changed to 29 per cent and 27 per cent respectively, but after state pension age the proportion who saw themselves as retired increased sharply to 86 per cent.

Self-definition as retired cannot be equated with lack of paid employment, especially for women. For women, the proportion defining themselves as retired also increased dramatically at state pension age, from 10 per cent of women in their late 50s to 51 per cent in their early 60s (Table 6.1). About a

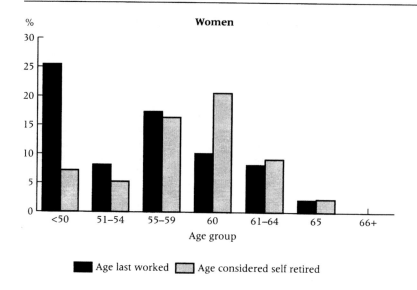

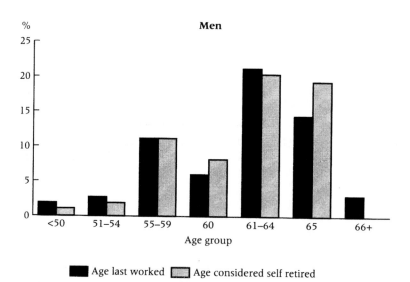

Figure 6.1   Age last employed and age retired, married women and men (aged 55–69)

Source: *Retirement and Retirement Plans Survey, 1988* (authors' analysis)

quarter of women over 60 described themselves as a housewife. The proportion was higher among women over 75, reflecting either a cohort difference in previous employment participation or in perceptions of gender roles. Only 60 per cent of women over 75 said they were retired, compared with virtually all men (97 per cent) at this age.

Passing the state pension age had a major influence on whether married women and men perceived themselves as retired, as shown in Figure 6.1. For men, the age of leaving their last job corresponded quite closely to the age when they considered themselves retired; at age 65, however, a higher proportion began to see themselves as retired than actually left their last job. For women, the disparity between these two measures and the impact of state pension age were more marked; before age 60, half of married women had left the labour market but only 28 per cent defined themselves as retired, while at state pension age only 10 per cent of women actually left their last job but 20 per cent said this was the age when they retired.

Thus research on retirement needs to distinguish between the age of last exit from paid employment and the self-defined age of retirement, especially when considering women's retirement. In analysing how partners time their retirement in relation to each other, we use the age of leaving last employment, since this is more significant to partners' relative income and to their gender roles.

Choice and constraint in the reasons for retirement

The concept of choice of retirement timing has limited relevance in Britain, as noted earlier. Table 6.2 shows the main reason why older married women and men left their last job, comparing those who left employment at different ages. Over half of married men had to leave because of their firm closing, redundancy, or health problems; such non-voluntary reasons were especially common among men who left employment before 60, reaching over 90 per cent for those leaving before 55. Among married women, a third left their last job for such non-voluntary reasons, as did half of those who left employment in their early 50s. A third of all women, and two-thirds of those who left before 50, did so for caring or family reasons. Such reasons may also be considered as non-voluntary insofar as they often represent caring for children or for a chronically sick spouse or older relative.

At state pension age, there is a marked rise in the proportion who report retirement as their reason for leaving. This suggests that for many people retirement from their job was mandatory at state pension age, and thus was not freely chosen. Therefore, the concept of choice of timing of last exit from employment is largely an inappropriate one among married women and men in Britain. Because of this we would expect to find less evidence of joint retirement and of patriarchal marital relations discouraging wives from working longer than husbands.

Table 6.2   Reason left last job by age left among not employed married women and men (aged 55–69)

(a) Married women

	Age left last job						
	≤50 %	51–4 %	55–9 %	60 %	61–4 %	65+ %	All %
Retired	3	12	30	83	68	84	31
Firm closure, redundancy	12	27	20	4	11	11	14
Ill-health, disability	17	23	24	6	12	5	17
Caring, family reasons	64	29	17	6	6	–	32
Other reasons	4	8	8	1	3	–	5
N =	309	96	203	119	100	19	846

(b) Married men

	Age left last job						
	≤50 %	51–4 %	55–9 %	60 %	61–4 %	65+ %	All %
Retired	–	7	20	49	43	91	43
Firm closure, redundancy	19	36	35	24	26	3	23
Ill-health, disability	76	55	37	24	26	5	29
Caring, family reasons	–	–	4	3	2	–	2
Other reasons	5	2	4	–	3	1	2
N =	37	44	161	71	205	138	656

Source: *Retirement and Retirement Plans Survey, 1988* (authors' analysis). In these tables some of the column percentages do not add up to 100 per cent because of rounding.

The employment patterns of older couples

Among couples, there are four possible combinations of employment status of partners: both employed, neither employed, the husband employed but not the wife (the traditional pattern), and the wife employed while her husband is not (the non-traditional pattern). Among couples in the Retirement Survey, where the wife was aged 55–69, 20 per cent were employed, falling from 42 per cent where wives were in their late 50s to 4 per cent where wives were a decade older (Table 6.3a). The proportions where neither was employed increased

Table 6.3   Employment status of married couples by age of wife

(a) Retirement Survey

| | Age of wife | | | All |
	55–59 %	60–64 %	65–69 %	55–69 %
Dual employed	42	11	4	20
Husband only employed	23	24	10	19
Wife only employed	13	10	5	10
Neither employed	22	55	81	51
N = (couples)	432	427	347	1206

Source: *Retirement and Retirement Plans Survey, 1988* (authors' analysis)

(b) General Household Survey

| | Age of wife | | | | | |
	40–44 %	45–49 %	50–54 %	55–59 %	60–64 %	65–69 %
Dual employed	73	71	57	39	13	4
Husband employed	19	17	22	23	22	12
Wife employed	3	5	10	13	8	3
Neither employed	4	7	11	25	57	81
N = (couples)	2321	1768	1622	1452	1380	1248

Source: *General Household Survey, 1988–90* (authors' analysis). In these tables some of the column percentages do not add up to 100 per cent because of rounding.

from 22 per cent to 81 per cent across this age range. In a fifth of couples, the husband alone was working, and in a tenth, the wife alone was working.

Although the pattern of a wife working while her husband is not goes against cultural norms about economic and social relationships between marital partners, this pattern occurred for 13 per cent of wives in their late 50s. Similar figures are found in the General Household Survey (1988–90), which has the advantage of a larger sample and a somewhat higher response rate (Table 6.3b). The comparability of data from these two surveys increases our confidence in the finding that among couples aged 55–69 where only one partner is employed, in about a third of the cases this is the wife.

The non-traditional pattern, where the wife alone was working, was much less common for wives under 50; it applied to only 5 per cent of wives in their late 40s, 3 per cent in their early 40s (Table 6.3b), and 2 per cent at younger ages (data not presented).

It seems likely that for younger couples, benefit regulations which involve wives' earnings being subject to a 'pound for pound' reduction in a family's Income Support have a substantial disincentive effect on women's employment. In mid-life, however, husbands who are not employed are more likely to have other sources of income, such as a pension and/or Invalidity Benefit and are less likely to rely solely on means tested benefits; there is then no financial penalty for women engaged in paid work. Our finding, that wives' sole employment was more common in mid-life than for younger couples, indicates that the influence of cultural norms against this non-traditional pattern may be somewhat less powerful than had been supposed from other studies (e.g. McKee 1987; Morris 1990). Alternatively, it may be that the cultural norms as to gender roles weaken after the childbearing phase of life.

Joint timing of employment exit among couples

This section explores the patterns of exit timing among older couples, excluding couples where both partners were still employed, since their future pattern of exit timing is unknown. We examine three patterns of exit timing among the remaining 81 per cent of couples. 'Joint exit' is defined as where partners left paid employment within six months of each other. The traditional pattern of exit applies where the husband left employment at least six months after his wife or was the sole earner at interview. The non-traditional pattern applies where the wife left her job at least six months after her husband, or she alone was employed at interview. Table 6.4 shows that among all couples for whom exit timing could be determined (row A), 60 per cent had followed the traditional pattern, 12 per cent the joint pattern, and 28 per cent the non-traditional pattern.

Thus the traditional pattern of the husband leaving the labour market after his wife is most common but in many cases this is because his wife left work much earlier in her life course, mainly because of childrearing. As shown in Table 6.2, women who left their last job before age 50 are unlikely to leave because of retirement.

In a third of the couples where exit timing could be determined, one or both partners left employment before age 51 (row B, Table 6.4). In most cases this was the wife, reflecting a traditional gendered pattern of employment where wives had left the labour market earlier in their life course, perhaps without re-entering employment after childbearing.

For a surprisingly large proportion of couples, two-thirds, both partners were employed at age 51 or later. If the analysis is restricted to these couples, the patterns of exit timing are much more evenly distributed: 43 per cent were traditional and 40 per cent non-traditional, with only 17 per cent leaving employment at around the same time (row C, Table 6.4). Where only one

Table 6.4 Work exit patterns of married couples (wife aged 55–69)

Employment pattern	% of couples	No. of couples	Traditional (husband later)	Joint exit pattern*	Non-traditional (wife later)	Row %
A All couples, excluding where both were employed at time of interview	100	976	60	12	28	100
B One or both partners stopped work before age 51	34	335	93	2	5	100
C Both partners stopped work at 51+	66	641	43	17	40	100
(i) Neither employed at interview	42	408	40	27	33	100
(ii) One partner only employed at interview	24	233	49	–	51	100

* 'Joint exit' is defined as employment exit of each partner within six months of each other.

Source: Retirement and Retirement Plans Survey, 1988 (authors' analysis)

Table 6.5   Exit patterns of couples by (a) reason wife left last job, (b) reason husband left last job (dual employed couples at age 51 or over)

(a) Wife's reason left last job

Exit pattern*	Retired %	Employers' actions[†] %	Ill-health/ Disability %	Caring/ family %	Other reason %	All %
Traditional (husband later)	45	57	67	49	53	52
Joint exit	23	23	12	20	12	20
Non-traditional (wife later)	32	20	21	32	35	28
N =	255	84	86	76	34	535
(%)	(48%)	(16%)	(16%)	(14%)	(6%)	(100%)

(b) Husband's reason left last job

Exit pattern*	Retired %	Employers' actions[†] %	Ill-health/ Disability %	Other reason %	All %
Traditional (husband later)	38	32	25	29	33
Joint exit	21	19	16	35	20
Non-traditional (wife later)	41	49	59	35	47
N =	276	131	118	14	542
(%)	(51%)	(24%)	(22%)	(3%)	(100%)

* Exit patterns exclude couples where both were employed at the time of interview. Joint refers to partners' exit within six months of each other.
[†] Employers' actions include redundancy, dismissal and firm closed down.

Source: Retirement and Retirement Plans Survey, 1988 (authors' analysis). In these tables some of the column percentages do not add up to 100 per cent because of rounding.

partner was employed at the time of interview, almost equal proportions of wives as husbands were sole employed (row C(ii)). These findings demonstrate considerable symmetry in exit timing among couples who were both employed in their early 50s.

We next consider how these three patterns of exit timing are related to partners' reasons for leaving their last job, restricting the analysis to couples where both partners were employed at age 51. Couples' patterns of exit timing are likely to depend on the degree of choice or constraint available to each partner, as indicated by the reason they left their last job. Table 6.5 shows that where one partner left for non-voluntary reasons, the other partner tended to remain employed longer, irrespective of gender. This gender symmetry is particularly noticeable for ill-health and disability; where a wife left for health reasons, in 67 per cent of couples the husband left later than his wife, compared with 45 per cent where the wife retired. Similarly, where a husband left for health reasons, in 59 per cent of couples the wife left later, compared with 41 per cent where the husband retired. Thus when a partner left because of ill-health, the other partner of either gender was likely to work longer. Where men left the labour market because of ill-health many wives continued in employment to provide what (in the US) has been called 'substitute' earnings.

We expect that joint exit is likely to be more difficult to achieve where wives or husbands retire for non-voluntary reasons, such as those stemming from employers' actions (mainly redundancy) or ill-health. Table 6.5 indicates that this is not so when employers' actions have precipitated exit. However, joint exit was least likely for those who left because of ill-health; only 16 per cent of husbands leaving for health reasons had joint exit and an even smaller proportion of wives, 12 per cent, were joined by their husbands. In some of these couples, one partner may have left employment at the same time as their spouse in order to care for them.

The traditional pattern of exit was most likely where the wife had left for non-voluntary reasons associated with employers' actions or ill-health, suggesting that this does not precipitate retirement of their husbands; but neither does husbands' exit for these reasons precipitate retirement of their wives. These findings suggest mainly symmetry in the influence of reasons for exit on the couple's exit pattern.

As discussed earlier, the cultural norm in most western societies, including Britain, is for men to marry women who are somewhat younger than themselves. This age asymmetry serves to reinforce patriarchal power in marriage, since the older partner tends initially to have greater financial resources and authority than the younger. The age difference between spouses would tend to lead to the non-traditional pattern of exit, were it not for the five year age difference in the state pension age of men and women, this facilitates exit timing which is either joint or traditional.

The way the age difference between partners influenced the couple's exit pattern is shown in Table 6.6. Wives who were much younger than their husband were more likely to leave later than their husband: 72 per cent where the wife was over 10 years younger and over half where she was between five and nine years younger. Where the wife was older than her husband or the same age, the traditional pattern of exit was followed by the majority of couples. The likelihood of joint exit varied little according to the age difference between partners, but was somewhat more likely where the wife was two to four years younger than her husband.

The polarization between the traditional and non-traditional patterns

Table 6.6   Exit patterns by age differential between spouses (couples both in paid employment at age 51 or later; wife aged 55–69)

Exit pattern*	Wife older		Same age† %	Wife younger			All %
	5+ yr %	2–4 yr %		2–4 yr %	5–9 yr %	10+ yr %	
Traditional (husband later)	80	68	56	45	20	12	43
Joint exit	13	14	13	21	18	16	17
Non-traditional (wife later)	7	18	31	34	62	72	40
N =	15	56	185	205	137	43	641
(%)	(2%)	(9%)	(29%)	(32%)	(21%)	(7%)	(100%)

* Exit patterns exclude couples where both were employed at the time of interview. 'Joint exit' refers to employment exit within six months of each other.
† Same age is defined as under 18 months age difference between partners.
Source: *Retirement and Retirement Plans Survey, 1988* (authors' analysis)

according to the age difference between spouses (Table 6.6) is consistent with symmetry in the effect of the age difference between partners, irrespective of the gender of the other partner, but it also reflects the effect of patriarchy enshrined in the earlier state pension age of women.

Conclusions

The age at which people consider themselves retired and the age when they leave their last job are only loosely related. This discrepancy is especially striking for married women in their 50s, when a substantial minority were neither employed, nor considered themselves to be retired. The state pension age had a marked influence on whether people said they were retired, irrespective of their actual employment status.

The influence of patriarchy is reflected in the proportion of older couples, 26 per cent, where the wife had left employment before she reached her 50s, mainly to perform a homemaking role. However, this pattern is now less common in Britain, since for nearly three-quarters of couples both partners were in employment at age 51 or above. Among these couples, there was near symmetry in the non-joint patterns of employment exit. The prevalence of constraints on individuals' freedom to choose when to leave their last job was likely to be the major reason for gender symmetry in exit timing among older couples. Most people left because of employer-related reasons, mandatory retirement or ill-health.

Only a small minority of British couples left their last jobs at about the same time. Such joint exits may be interpreted as reflecting choice in retirement timing. However, joint retirement may also signify involuntary exit by one partner triggering exit by the other.

The age difference between partners is important in exit timing. The non-traditional pattern, where the wife continued to work after her husband had retired, was more common where the wife was five or more years younger than her husband. This suggests that retirement timing of couples is sensitive to such factors as when each partner reaches state pension age and that the traditional pattern is reinforced by unequal state pension ages in combination with the marriage age differential.

The intention of the British government to raise the pension age for women to 65, phasing in the change from the year 2010 (HMSO 1994) is likely to have implications for the retirement timing of couples. Women will need an extra five years' National Insurance contributions or credits in order to be eligible for a full state basic pension, but if they retire at age 65, this will usually be after their husbands' retirement. To the extent that there are pressures to avoid contravening the norm of male economic dominance, in addition to lack of employment opportunities, wives will continue to retire well before the new state pension age of 65, thus reducing their chance of fulfilling eligibility requirements for a full state pension as well as the value of any other pensions.

If married women continue to leave the labour market mainly in their late 50s, the gap between their retirement and pension age will be widened, making the majority of wives wholly financially dependent on their husbands until age 65. If there are no changes in the opportunities for employment for older women, raising the state pension age to 65 will mean women will find it more difficult than at the present time to acquire sufficient pension rights to ensure their financial well-being in later life. Thus although the legislative change will provide incentives for women to remain in employment until 65, its main effect is likely to be penalizing women for leaving the labour market before 65.

We conclude that constraints associated with the lack of opportunities for both men and women in the labour market in their 50s and early 60s have a major impact on the pattern of couples' exit timing. Our research suggests that cultural norms which militate against women being in paid employment when their husbands are not working are much weaker among older couples than they are at earlier stages of the life course.

In conclusion, both gender role symmetry among couples employed in their 50s and feminist theory contribute to explaining couples' retirement timing. There is greater symmetry than at earlier stages of the life course, for example, with each partner likely to continue in employment after the other leaves because of ill-health. Older employed women's choices are constrained mainly by factors operating in the labour market, but there is also evidence that the traditional pattern of exit timing predominates.

Acknowledgements

For access to the OPCS Retirement and Retirement Plans Survey and the General Household Survey data for 1988–1992 we are indebted to the ESRC Data Archive, University of Essex (OPCS 1988–92), and to the University of Manchester Computer Centre. We are grateful to the Office of Population Censuses and Surveys for permission to use these datasets. The chapter is based on a research project funded by the Economic and Social Research Council (Grant No. R000233240).

7

THE MARRIED LIVES OF OLDER PEOPLE

Janet Askham

The marital relationships of older people commonly merit two or three paragraphs in social gerontological textbooks and often barely one in sociological books on marriage and the family; perhaps they are considered unproblematic, even uninteresting. This chapter analyses why there may be such a view, and argues that the married lives of older people are of great interest and importance.

Despite increasing research attention old age is still frequently viewed as outside the mainstream of sociological theorizing and investigation. This has affected the study of many aspects of later life, including that of marriage, resulting in a restricted range of research questions, often of a narrowly gerontological kind. One reason suggested for the neglect of later life is that the explanatory frameworks of sociologists have traditionally centred on work (Kohli 1988; Arber and Ginn 1991b). Societies have been seen as work-orientated, and work has been the root of systems of social inequality, values, norms and the development of identities. However, argues Kohli, population ageing makes a fundamental difference; in a society in which a large proportion of the population has left the workforce, ageing must be a concern of mainstream sociological study with 'a more encompassing conception of age and the life course as a general dimension of social structure' (Kohli 1988: 369). One of the basic relationships retained by most people after they lose the fundamental one of employment is that of marriage; this is one of the reasons why marriage is an important element in theoretical developments now, when an unprecedented proportion of the population is retired.

Other developments in modern western society (which are often referred to as postmodernity) also necessitate moving some aspects of sociological study from the wings to centre stage. Bauman (1992) for example has argued that sociology needs a new focus of enquiry appropriate to the postmodern age. Postmodernity encompasses developments such as the decline of religious and moral traditions; the continuous examining and revising of meaning and values by the individual (reflexivity) which generates insecurity and doubt; and the relegation of much social behaviour and relationships to the private rather than the public sphere, thus removing them from public scrutiny and from the constraints of community norms. For example, it has been argued that death, once a public event, has been increasingly confined within the private sphere because it challenges 'an individual's consciousness of what is meaningful and real' (Mellor 1993: 27); by apparently negating individuality, death challenges a fundamental value of postmodernity. Death is a very important area of study because 'if we can understand the modern approach to death we can understand a great deal about modern society in general' (Mellor 1993: 24–25). Also within the private sphere are relationships such as marriage. The latter, however, far from challenging postmodern values, provides the clearest expression of such values. Within marriage, traditional values and norms are breaking down, leaving individuals to use the relationship to construct and maintain their own sense of identity and security. This change has been described as one from marriage as an institution to marriage as a relationship. A postmodern sociology must therefore increasingly be concerned with how a sense of personal meaning, identity and security are developed and maintained and with behaviour or relationships within the private sphere. Because of their central position in postmodern society such relationships should not be peripheral but should be part of mainstream study.

Thus the study of marriage in later life has been neglected for two reasons: first, because it is concerned with the lives of a group of the population seen as marginal to society's mainstream projects, and second, because it is seen as part of the private sphere and, therefore, as not forming part of the major sociological explanatory framework. The arguments of theorists like Kohli and Mellor demonstrate that it is time the marriages of older people in postmodern society were included in mainstream study. Older people, who in the public sphere are mainly consumers rather than producers, should receive attention in a world where people's consumption patterns are just as valid indicators of their position in society as their role in production; and marriage, although it is increasingly seen as beyond the public gaze, is a particularly important relationship in later life when the social relationships associated with employment have been lost. If the private sphere is pertinent to sociological study then this must include later life marriages.

The study of later life marriage may benefit from the recent theorizing and research about marriage in earlier life, which has burgeoned as a result of growing attention to the private sphere. This chapter aims to discuss how such research can illuminate later life marriage. It is useful, first, to provide a summary of sociological knowledge about marriage in later life.

Marriage relationships in later life

The paucity of British research on the topic of marriage in later life is revealed in an edited British volume on *Marriage, Domestic Life and Social Change* (Clark 1991a). The book was able to cite only one reference to recent British research specifically on later life marriage (Mason 1987). Most research on such relationships emanates from the USA (Brubaker 1990) and is mainly limited to studies of marital satisfaction or the division of domestic responsibilities. For the purposes of this chapter the term 'marriage' is used to refer mainly to the relationship between legally married heterosexual couples, and mainly to long term marriages rather than to those contracted in later life.

On the issue of marital satisfaction, it appears that most people are happy with their marriages, though older men have been found to be more satisfied than older women (Quirouette and Gold 1992). Although findings are mixed, the majority view appears to be that satisfaction with marriage improves with age after the nadir of the middle years when the couple was preoccupied with childrearing and careers, but that satisfaction may decline somewhat in very late life when increased frailty sets in (Lupri and Frideres 1981; Anderson *et al.* 1983; Gilford 1984). However there appears to be no direct relationship of marital satisfaction with either retirement (Atchley 1992) or physical frailty (Johnson 1985). In fact there is no clear evidence about what factors influence the level of satisfaction, apart from the adverse effect of mental illness in one of the spouses (Wright 1991) and the positive effects of continued sexual activity with the spouse and social interaction with friends (Lee 1988; Ade-Ridder 1990). Satisfaction with the marriage does not appear to be affected by such events as adult children having problems or the physical health of one's spouse and in general it seems to stand up well to the vicissitudes of later life.

Studies of this kind, however, may conceal important variations; when finer distinctions are made between groups, different results may emerge. For example, researchers who examined the effects of a spouse's retirement found that wives' employment status does not appear to affect husbands but that having a retired husband significantly reduced wives' marital satisfaction (Lee and Shehan 1989).

Being married appears to be beneficial for people in later life, particularly for men (Mouser *et al.* 1985); married people live longer, have higher life satisfaction or morale, better mental and physical health, higher economic resources, more social support and lower rates of admission to institutions. However, the causal direction is not certain, since being healthy and happy may promote longevity and stable relationships.

Turning to the division of household and domestic responsibilities, it appears that the division of tasks among current older couples conforms to traditional gender roles, with men doing a few more tasks, mainly masculine ones, after their retirement and women continuing with the feminine tasks (Rexroat and Shehan 1987; Cliff 1993). This pattern changes somewhat as couples enter very late life, with men increasingly helping with traditionally feminine tasks.

Such changes have been found to have a negative effect upon wives' – though not husbands' – psychological well-being (Keith and Wacker 1990). Among those younger couples where the husband takes part in traditionally feminine tasks, however, these negative effects seem absent, suggesting that such couples will enter later life with quite different expectations from today's older couples. Some would argue that the main bases of the division of responsibility do not change in retirement, but that there is 'a repatterning of what those responsibilities mean in practice' (Mason 1987: 93). There is no clear evidence about what factors influence any change in the division of domestic responsibilities, though the physical or mental frailty of either spouse seems to do so (see Chapter 8 by Wilson and Chapter 9 by Rose and Bruce).

This brief summary of research on marital relationships in later life (discussed more fully in Askham 1994) shows that there are many areas about which little is known. Nor can we assume that the evidence from the USA is applicable to Britain. There are serious methodological difficulties about much of the research; in particular, there is almost no research on older people's own perceptions of the meaning of marriage. Most research does not take the perspective of the couple or the relationship itself, but only of the individual within that relationship. For example, information about wives is rarely analysed in relation to information about their husbands; and the extent and nature of the interaction between them is not often the subject of attention, particularly by means of observation. Almost no attention has been given to variations among different groups of married people, for example by ethnicity or financial resources, or to groups such as the very old, the disabled, or the unhappily married.

The focus on marital satisfaction and the division of domestic responsibilities has diverted attention away from other dimensions of marriage, such as other sources of commitment to the relationship, other services which the spouses may perform for each other, or other possessions or activities which they may share. It may be instructive to think about why there has been such an emphasis upon these two elements in later life marriages. The research interest in marital satisfaction accords with the view of marriage as a private relationship rather than a public institution by implying that what is important, and what holds a marriage together, is how the spouses feel about each other and about their relationship. This is despite some evidence that feelings about each other are less likely to be what sustains a marriage in later life than in earlier life; the weight of investment the partners have made in the relationship and their shared history may take precedence (Reedy *et al.* 1981; Johnson 1985). In one sense, a long term relationship is very firmly in the public sphere; the sheer number of occasions on which it has been publicly acknowledged is obviously likely to be greater than for more recent marriages (even though much of the daily lives of older couples, as suggested earlier in this chapter, is likely to be hidden from public gaze).

Research on marital satisfaction may also be seen to treat the marriage as private in that it avoids asking for intimate details; it does not 'pry' too deeply into the relationship, merely assessing how satisfied people are with it or with various aspects of it. It would be interesting to find out in what contexts we ask people in our everyday lives about how happy or satisfied they are; it may be for example that this is something we are particularly likely to ask of children rather than adults, or that it is culturally specific, perhaps being more of a preoccupation in the USA than in Britain. There is indeed evidence that people in the USA are more likely than the British to believe that the married are happier than the unmarried (Jowell *et al.* 1990: 62).

The preoccupation with marital satisfaction seems to treat marriage as a variable rather than as a topic of interest in its own right. The intention is to summarize the complexity of each marriage through an assessment of satisfaction, in order to examine how other factors vary by this summary marital satisfaction measure.

The reason for the interest in the division of household responsibilities – the other main topic of investigations of later life marriages – is probably different. Much of the research does centre on marriage itself, but (with exceptions such as Mason 1987) it has been more concerned with who actually performs each task rather than with the power balance within the relationship – that is, who has the authority or responsibility or final say in decisions. This focus on tasks may be because the interest is not so much sociological as social policy driven, springing from a desire to know to what extent couples can cope when one or both become frail or disabled, or it may be to do with the difficulty of obtaining valid measures of power, whereas data on task performance is more readily available. Although much of the recent research on the domestic division of labour appears pedestrian, it has an interesting history, originating in the highly influential work of Bott (1957) which showed how joint and segregated marriages were related to the characteristics of the couple's social network. Where research on task division is also concerned with social networks, it is less confined to the private realm than is research on marital satisfaction.

To understand why so many dimensions and concerns of later life marriage have been ignored it is helpful to review recent research on the sociology of marriage more generally.

Theory and areas of study in recent sociological research on marriage

Theoretical issues

There has been considerable theoretical interest in marriage (see Morgan 1985). The theoretical perspectives which have had most influence are:

- symbolic interactionism. This approach has emphasized the importance in modern western societies of the intimate relationship and the interaction within it for developing and maintaining people's sense of personal identity (Askham 1984).

- feminist theory. This has been important for its examination of the relationship between the sexes in marriage and for its stress upon the patriarchal structures and values which reinforce some traditional forms of marriage and the subservience of wives (Gittins 1985).
- structuralist theoretical approaches concerned with the analysis of the course of late capitalist society. Ways in which elements of late capitalism have affected or will affect marriage behaviour have been suggested. For example, increasing technological and bureaucratic control makes people less able to exert control, even in areas of life where they might be thought to have the choice (such as marriage); the increasing importance of the market and of consumption as opposed to production requires that women and men develop as separate markets, and this increasingly drives a wedge between women and men. The resulting gender conflict of interest is likely to discourage joint action and to contribute to high divorce rates. In addition, it may be suggested that the market encourages divorce because serial marriage requires greater consumption of houses, furnishings, weddings and so on.

Analysis of the pressures on the state and public policies also involves theorizing about marriage. Here one can see some of the contradictions which marriages may be facing, for the pressures emanating from statutory provisions look rather different from those of the market. Governments concerned to cut welfare spending emphasize family care, thus placing a heavy reliance on marriage; marriages are asked to bear as much as possible of the care of dependent spouses, children and parents; and the state must encourage marriages to endure in order to curtail the number of ex-spouses with care needs or emotional needs (Department of Health 1989).

Theoretical interests, therefore, span a wide range. The same is true of the specific themes or topics of empirical study in recent years.

Empirical research

Interaction between spouses in the early stages of marriage has received some research attention. This stems from interest in the social construction of the marital relationship, for example the scope for negotiation couples have over forms of marriage, and the development and maintenance of the sense of identity within intimate relationships. Studies have shown that there is considerable variation among couples in the nature of their current relationship and in their approach to the future. For example, Mansfield and Collard (1988), in a study of newly married couples, found three types of orientation to the future among couples: the 'planners', 'venturers' and 'roamers'. The planners had a strong sense of direction and clear ideas about where they were going and who they were going to be. The venturers had broad strategies but few specific plans; they placed more emphasis on chance and luck but were generally optimistic and forward looking. The roamers had 'neither plans nor strategies' and appeared to take life as it came. In a study of both first and subsequent marriages Clark (1982, 1991b) similarly identified people with a relatively weak orientation to the future (drifters), others whose current or future views and plans were influenced by the past ('surfacers' and to some extent 'strugglers'), those who were influenced by external factors ('strugglers' again) and those with clear plans for a future ('establishers'). Scope for variation is there, but it is not unlimited; there are very strong influences from the outside world, such as economic circumstances or the influence of previous spouses or others.

One of the most important additional findings from Mansfield and Collard (1988) (and one which can be found in many other studies) was the great difference between wives and husbands in their experience and perception of marriage, with wives giving their jobs less priority after marriage and taking on more of the household responsibilities than husbands, and placing more emphasis on communication and sharing than the men. Studies of the unequal distribution of resources and power in marriage have been pursued through, for example, research on housework and childcare or on the process of marital breakdown (Clark 1987; Henwood *et al.* 1987). There has also been some attention to the handling of money in marriage (Pahl 1989; 1990) and how this is related to financial decision making.

Internal conflicts, pressures and threats to the marriage have been explored in studies which follow on from the early stage of marriage relationships and examine marriages in mid-course. These have shown some of the internal contradictions of the relationship; for example, Askham (1984) identified a conflict between the search for a sense of identity and for a sense of security or stability within marriage, but found that couples were often very successful in steering a middle course and developing a compromise between the two.

The external threats to a couple's relationship, such as children, adultery, unemployment or poverty, have received much less attention than they warrant, though there has been some relatively recent interest (see for example, Lawson 1988, on adultery; and McKee and Bell 1985, on marriage and unemployment). This relative lack of interest is probably due to the increasing emphasis upon the 'private ordering of family life' (Clulow 1991: 168) as opposed to institutional regulation and external influences. But paradoxically the appreciation of the 'private ordering' of marriage has given rise (along with feminist pressure) in recent years to an interest in the risk of psychological or physical damage to the individual within marriage. For example, discussion of marital rape, and physical or mental abuse is beginning (Smith 1989; Dobash and Dobash 1992; Whittaker, Chapter 11). The prevailing ideologies of marriage may still uphold the long term heterosexual couple relationship as a good thing, but there is increasing recognition that it may be bad for women and even for men in certain circumstances (Delphy and Leonard 1992).

Attention is increasingly being devoted to change in marriage and intimate relationships. The major change is, as stated above, that marriage is moving from 'institution' to 'relationship.' For example particular historical periods have been examined and the influence of institutional, political or value change on marital behaviour assessed (see for instance Finch and Summerfield 1991). Such studies usually evaluate change (or lack of it) in marriage in different cohorts rather than in individual marriages. As with studies of marriage in later life, there is very little longitudinal investigation. In this area, theoretical development and hypotheses suggest more change in marriage than is supported by research evidence. Thus Finch and Summerfield (1991) suggest that postwar changes added to the strain on wives through imposing yet more responsibilities rather than bringing about a more equal relationship as argued by Young and Willmott (1973). During the postwar period: 'In addition to the demands that a wife should be more comradely, more motherly, more sensuous, and a better homemaker, was added the expectation that she should be a part-time wage earner' (Finch and Summerfield 1991: 17). It should be remembered, however, that despite evidence of the continuation of women's multiple roles, with the strain that that implies, there is also evidence that women who are employed are happier than housewives with similar characteristics, due to the sense of identity and the companionship gained from paid work outside the home (Sharpe 1984).

The fact that observed change between cohorts in marriage is less than expected may be due partly, as Giddens says, to 'institutional lag', in which institutions preserve an appearance of stability even after their functions have been largely lost or changed:

> Heterosexual marriage superficially appears to retain its central position in the social order . . . In reality, it has been largely undermined by the rise of the pure relationship and plastic sexuality. If orthodox marriage is not yet widely seen as just one life-style among others, as in fact it has become, this is partly the result of institutional lag and partly the result of the complicated mixture of attraction and repulsion which the psychic development of each sex creates with regard to the other.
>
> (1992: 154)

There has indeed been considerable research interest in newer forms of intimate relationship, though they do not yet appear to have the same standing in public perception as marriage or cohabitation. We are now experiencing a second wave of interest in 'deviant' forms of relationship; in the 1970s there was an interest in communal living, wifeswapping and so on. This was followed in the 80s and 90s by an interest in lesbian and gay relationships, as well as in the much more common incidence of second or subsequent marriages (see Burgoyne and Clark 1984; Clark 1987).

Finally, there has been some attention to ideologies of marriage. By this is meant how marriage is portrayed in publicly available accounts and in popular beliefs as to what marriage is and should be like. The ideological elements which Morgan (1991) sees as increasingly stressed by professionals (and probably increasingly embodied in lay thinking) are: marriage as the paramount relationship, freely chosen, based on love, and for the benefit of the individual; marriage as a provider of security and a means of stabilizing life's trajectories (though this may conflict with its role as an open and spontaneous relationship within which personal growth can take place). This is a very positive ideology offering to satisfy widely felt but conflicting needs – those of freedom and security; it is also portrayed as having general applicability. As Morgan says, it does not emphasize differences between men and women, or ethnic or class groups. So it papers over differences and helps in the construction of a communal sense of identity.

Application to later life marriages

Returning to older people one can ask how the above developments can aid understanding of marital relationships in later life. First, on a theoretical level, they suggest that studies of later life marriages are lagging far behind studies concerned with earlier stages of the life course. An interactionist perspective on later life marriage is largely lacking (see below). Feminist theory is beginning to take an interest in older women, but at present this is mainly through attention to caring responsibilities for frail family members; older women's other disadvantages in marriage, in terms of domestic responsibilities, financial position and decision making power also need attention. Structuralist theories of late capitalism have not been applied to questions of marriage in later life. One might suggest that with the increased needs of the economic system for consumption, postmodern society would require older couples to be optimistic about the future and ignore the prospect of death because only thus would they want to go on consuming new goods and replacing old ones (see Martin 1990; Bury, Chapter 2). It would also encourage older couples to stay together because with their lower incomes they are a more viable consumption unit as a couple than as single households. Although the economy may benefit from divorce at younger ages, this is less likely to apply when the chance of remarriage and rebuilding a home lessens in later life. Marital stability is also needed to provide care, either mutual or unilateral, with the decline in the state's role as provider of such services. Theoretical considerations suggest therefore that modern older marriages, like younger marriages, are important to society but are subject to considerable strain.

Research on orientations to the future in earlier marriage show that couples come to later life marriage from a variety of different starting points, and that these are influenced by both individual values, internal negotiation or construction, and external factors. Some older husbands and wives will have been planners, some venturers, drifters, roamers and so on. The satisfaction of plans fulfilled may be all that is needed by former planners; or their habit of planning may require the same approach at a stage where planning may be more difficult because of likely short trajectories, unknown time of onset of frailty or death and inability to control their financial situation.

Studies of gender differences suggest that in later life as in earlier there will be the man's and the woman's marriage (Bernard 1976). Does a patriarchal system maintain the husband's advantageous position or are there counter-vailing forces in later life when the husband no longer has a position in the labour force? In terms of income, men's earlier advantage is transmitted into later life through their higher pensions; they remain financially dominant over their wives (Ginn and Arber 1991). Do men's physical advantages disappear? Does men's tendency to dominance diminish at the same time as psychological changes in their wives (see Gutmann 1987) encourage the latter to become more dominant and forceful? Despite the mass of research on division of household responsibilities in later life we still have no clear answers to these questions. However, the chapters by Rose and Bruce and by Wilson begin to answer them.

Studies of prevailing ideologies of marriage do not specifically discuss older people's marriages, although they assume general applicability. How does the change in marriage from institution to relationship affect older people? Are they too changing? Are their views influenced more by current fashions, by the age they have reached or by the historical time which they and the rest of their cohort have lived through over the years? If older people's views are primarily derived from the past, do they feel out of step with views which reflect the prevailing national identity? And if so, how do they react to this disparity (Coleman and McCulloch 1985)? Are their marriages more institution than relationship? If so, is this because they married at a time when marriage was more closely defined by social norms, or because the marriage has through its own longevity become routine? Because it is accepted nowadays that unhappy marriages break up, can the low divorce rate of older couples be seen as a sign of their happiness? (In 1991 the 25 to 29 age group in England and Wales showed the highest rate of divorce, at 33 per thousand of the married population; the rate for those aged 45 and over was only 5.6 per thousand (Central Statistical Office 1994).) But it may be that there are other reasons why marriages last, such as traditional views or lack of positive advantages in divorcing at older ages.

Studies which have looked particularly at interaction within marriage and at the internal contradictions or conflicts have little to say about later life marriages. However, it is implied that the conversation, the reflexivity which permits people to develop and maintain a sense of identity continues into old age. We know very little about it, however. The opportunities for physical or psychological harm to one's spouse are certainly as likely in older as in younger marriages (see Whittaker, Chapter 11). Such abuse may be particularly likely when one member becomes frail or when there is no one else to have power over (as children have left and subordinates at work are a thing of the past). It may not be the frail member who loses power however; the carer may be the subservient one, especially now that he or she has to do so much for the other partner. Rose and Bruce (Chapter 9) suggest that even physically dependent men frequently retain power over their wives.

The influence of various external factors upon marital satisfaction in later life has been examined but comparatively little is known about how they are experienced, or about how they may affect other aspects of the marital relationship. For example, very little is known about how poverty affects later life marital relationships.

Finally, what about the changing forms of marriage? Is it the case that older people feel freer to enter new kinds of relationships, such as gay or lesbian partnerships, or to espouse them as normal? There has been some research on gay relationships among older people, and there is little suggestion that they are generally becoming more acceptable, though there may be some attempts to accommodate changing views. As Giddens says:

> In contrast to those in younger age groups today the experience of older women was almost always framed in terms of marriage, even if the person in question did not marry . . . Marriage was to them the core experience of a woman's life – although many have had retrospectively to reconstruct their past because, when they first got married, marriage was very different from what it is now.
>
> (1992: 53)

Looking again at the two main areas of research on later life marriage, marital satisfaction studies begin to look very old fashioned in the light of the recent theoretical and empirical investigations into marital interaction. The time has come to develop more sophisticated models of marriage and the activities and processes which take place in the relationship. Studies of the division of household responsibilities look less outdated but need to be more directly informed by theoretical concerns about power and authority within marriage, and to look more fully at areas of activity hitherto not studied in any detail in later life, such as money or decision making or activities beyond those of domestic tasks. Most importantly, time and change themselves should be the focus of attention. As different cohorts of married people enter old age, and as old age itself changes within the postmodern world, urgent questions about how older couples experience marriage remain to be answered.

8

'I'M THE EYES AND SHE'S THE ARMS': CHANGES IN GENDER ROLES IN ADVANCED OLD AGE

Gail Wilson

There are now many more people of *advanced* old age in society than there have ever been before (Eekelaar and Pearl 1989). This new age group has not yet been socially constituted as a separate life stage. There is a mismatch between negative social expectations of old age and reality. The space created may allow women a new freedom in the way gender relations and gender identities can be constructed in advanced old age. This chapter draws on the experience of men and women over 75 to show how some women are able to take advantage of the change even though most are still restricted by poverty, ill health (their own or their partner's) and patriarchal beliefs.

The concept of advanced old age is intended as a term which is meaningful to older people at a certain stage in the life course rather than any specific chronological age. Advanced years are an essential ingredient, but there can be no specific threshold or set of characteristics which determine individual classifications. There is a need, as Bury (Chapter 2) says, to distinguish macro and micro levels of categorization and experience. The micro involves personal and social experience. At the personal level, length of life implies a mix of experiences which can be categorized as specific to the person concerned, and also experiences which are personal but which relate to the individual's social position. Social position in advanced old age may be defined in terms of family or friends and expressed in terms of descendants – grandchildren and great-grandchildren in the direct line, or great-nieces and nephews or more distant relatives. Those without a position in a blood line still have the ability to look back and see themselves as part of a series of different social networks. Individuals may also identify themselves as having lived through, or as continuing to live in, a range of social groupings with separate or interlocking histories. Insofar as a definition of advanced old age is possible, the intention is to convey that life has been long, that much has been experienced and that the inevitability of death is either acknowledged or subliminally present.

Advanced old age, therefore, from the point of view of older people themselves, implies very much more than the passage of time. The term is less clearly definable from the point of view of younger generations. They may make few distinctions among 'the old' and may see men and women aged from 70 to 90 as much the same. Ageism is strong in western society (Stearns 1977; Bytheway 1995) and the 'old' are frequently stereotyped as frail, certainly physically, and probably mentally too.

The ageist stereotypes manifested by the majority of the younger generation and the internalization of attitudes to age acquired during the life course, result in age becoming the key defining characteristic of later life. Men and women are seen as 'old' before they are characterized in any other way. This does not mean that age is the great leveller, wiping out class, race and gender differences, but it means that other attributes take second place to age as the key influence on social identity and social relationships in the way people in advanced old age are categorized by others. This is true of social identity even though many older people will say that they do not *feel* old (Itzin 1990b).

Some have argued that there is a positive side to ageism as well as a negative. Constraints may be relaxed because 'the old' are not thought capable. For example 'when you reach a certain age, if they don't like what you say, they think you're a bit batty anyway, so you get away with it' (quoted in Nicholson 1980: 228). In other words there are opportunities which come from social marginalization as well as costs.

In this chapter, gender and ageing are considered within a framework that takes account of age (chronological, physiological and social, see Chapter 1), stage in the life course, cohort and period effects. A life course approach to ageing has the advantage that 'it eschews a static view of old age in isolation, providing a dynamic framework which focuses on change and continuity' (Arber and Evandrou 1993: 10). It also avoids the use of chronological cut-off points, such as pension age, or age 75 (the threshold age for annual general practitioner health checks).

However, life course effects are not the only influences on gender relations in advanced old age. Both cohort (or generation) effects and secular changes (or period effects) have to be considered. The men and women discussed in this chapter were born between 1896 and 1916 – before and during World War I. They can therefore be seen as making up two cohorts (with some overlap), one that reached their teens before or during the war and another which grew up during the interwar depression. The impact of belonging to these cohorts varies among individuals and among classes but can be identified as a series of group phenomena.

For many women in the study, the most salient cohort effect was the loss of men during World War I. The unusually high number of never married women is partly accounted for by a lack of partners (see Table 8.1). These women had fulfilled gendered roles in their families in the past, as daughters and carers for sisters, aunts and parents, but had now ceased to do so. They had also, in nearly all cases, had to work for a living throughout most of their lives. In advanced old age some continued to cook and clean, but others had long ago given up cooking. For men the experience of unemployment or job insecurity in the interwar depression had a major influence on their life course. This was true for most middle-class as well as all working-class men.

Secular or period effects refer to changes which have an impact on all age groups in a society at any one time, rather than on any specific cohort. Rising prosperity and greater educational and employment opportunities for women were period effects identified by members of the study cohorts.

Gender relations and gender identities observed in advanced old age today are the product of the interaction between individual life courses and cohort and period effects. However, this chapter argues that the main influence is the rise of a new phase of life (Rosenmayr 1982), which is identified by the numbers now attaining it, but not by any socially prescribed way of living. Generations need a 'rehearsal time' to adjust to new social structures (Bengtson 1989). As Riley says, 'for the greatly expanded numbers of people in the oldest ages, too few new roles have so far been institutionalised . . . Older women in particular . . . are in the end the ones most often left alone to create new roles for themselves' (1985: 339).

The assumptions behind the following discussion of gender in later life are that gender has both material and non-material aspects, and is affected in different ways by changes in a range of social spheres. In economic terms, gender relations are affected by changes in levels of income in a society and by changes in the distribution of income between men and women. Economic conditions are related to social conditions, but changes in these also have their own effects on gender identities and gender relations. Work opportunities, housing, education, transport and personal safety have an interactive influence on gender relations. Dominant ideologies, particularly of the family and the capacities of women and men, have long term effects on the way individuals think about themselves and the way society relates to them. Religious and other beliefs constitute another set of influences. Personal relations, beliefs about self-identity, family relations and individual life events affect the way men and women speak about gender relations, how they act and how closely they relate discourse and action.

It is possible to argue that the patterns of gender relations described in this chapter are a cause of long life rather than a consequence of it. Virtually all those interviewed were survivors in that they had passed the average age of death. If autonomy is helpful in maintaining well-being, and in putting off mortality, as proponents of holistic medicine argue (Scrutton 1992), then it is to be expected that there will be a higher survival rate among women and men who are able to live more autonomous lives. The sample were more healthy physically and mentally than the average for the locality in terms of physical and mental health. One ingredient in their survival may have been their ability to exercise autonomy in gender relations and in the ways they constituted gendered identity in later life.

Method

The aim of the study was to investigate daily living among people over the age of 75 in an outer London borough. Two wards with contrasting socioeconomic status were chosen. In both, more than 20 per cent of the population were over retirement age in 1981. The sample was drawn from a survey of every fifth household consisting only of people over 75. The sample included Jewish refugees from Europe but no other ethnic minority elders. Recent migrants had not reached the lower age limit.

The areas were chosen to reflect likely national patterns of future family support. Neither ward formed part of a close-knit multi-generational community, since many of the younger generation had moved away. Distances varied, but the majority of respondents had no relatives within easy walking distance. The patterns of gender relations recorded are likely to have been affected by this, since the presence of family seemed to encourage men and women to maintain stereotypical divisions of labour when they might otherwise have taken on new activities. In the working-class ward, children and grandchildren had frequently bettered themselves and neighbouring homes were occupied by recent migrants, many from overseas. In the more prosperous ward, house prices had risen greatly. The few elders who had children living locally had moved into the area to be near their high income children. Others were long term residents but their families were scattered.

Both areas were similar in terms of town planning, with a few large roads, fairly steep hills, quiet culs-de-sac and peripheral shopping parades. Neither had any public houses but both had several churches. Housing was almost entirely two storey with gardens front and back. Privet hedges and lawns caused similar problems of maintenance to frail older people in both areas. The need for assistance with gardens was therefore above the national average and the question of who did the gardening was a material one.

The study involved three rounds of interviews. First round interviews were conducted in a total of 94 households, 38 in the working-class area and 55 in the more prosperous area in 1991. Table 8.1 shows the initial composition of the households in the sample. The age range was from 75–96. Refusal rates at first interview were high, 48 per cent in the working-class area and 33 per cent in the better-off area. Such high refusal rates are normal in London (Bowling *et al.* 1992). A comparison between households which refused and those which took part showed that people who refused were in poorer physical and mental health than those who participated. The sample is therefore biased in favour of elders who are healthy. In the second round, 57 households were interviewed; the loss was mainly caused by deaths. A further 16 per cent were not

Table 8.1   Household composition of people interviewed in round one

| | Marital status | | | | |
	Married	Widowed	Separated	Single	Total
Men	31	8	2	1	42
Women	31	37	1	14	89*
Total households	31	45	3	15	94

* Includes two households with a married couple and single woman, two households with two widows, one household with two never married women and one household with a never married man and his mother.

interviewed in the third round mainly because of death or very serious ill health. Four years separate first and last interview rounds. In the first round respondents were asked about their arrangements for daily living, using a semi-structured interview schedule. In the second round they were asked about their health and financial arrangements, using a mixture of structured and semi-structured questions. The third round concentrated on views of the role of pensioners, the position of women, self-image and elder abuse.

Qualitative methods were used for two reasons. First, very little is known about normal ageing in the community in advanced old age, and the aim was to give elders a voice and to allow them to take charge of the interviews to some degree. Second, there are ethical problems in attempting to use standardized questionnaires in interviews with people who may be frail, either physically or mentally, who are possibly distressed by recent bereavement (not un-common), and who may not wish to answer questions on subjects such as money, sex or family relations. No one was excluded from the sample on the ground of mental frailty. Interviewers gave priority to the wishes of the respondent over the collection of standardized data. For example, household members determined who was interviewed. In some households only the husband was interviewed, in some the wife, and in others both were present for all or part of the interview and participation varied between rounds. Throughout the interviews respondents were encouraged to talk about issues that mattered to them.

Transcribed interviews were analysed using a computerized data processing package (Nud*ist; Richards *et al.* 1992). This programme allows lines or blocks of text to be grouped under themes or concepts. The blocks can be arranged in 'trees' or reassembled in different ways which may emerge as important during data processing. The aim was to group the words of men and women as they related to a range of activities and concepts associated with gender relations. The first of these were stereotypical divisions of labour in the areas of cooking, cleaning, gardening, management of money, leisure interests and activities.

The second were concerned with sexuality and attitudes to gender roles and relationships.

The link between age and gender is extremely complex. The research reported in this chapter represents a preliminary investigation of some aspects of the relationship between gender and ageing. It is limited in scope but also in time and place. Other societies constitute old age differently and can therefore be expected to produce different gendered patterns in later life.

Public and private accounts

Statements or views are unlikely to be exact descriptions of behaviour or action. They may not even be consistently held or believed. Cornwell (1984) drew attention to public and private accounts, noting that public accounts tend to be those most likely to be publicly acceptable and to represent a socially approved stereotype. Private accounts may differ or conflict with public accounts. Cornwell noted that her respondents had no difficulty in offering conflicting accounts of health beliefs or life chances in the same or different interviews. Areas such as gender relations, where there is a dominant ideology which may bear little relationship to direct experience, are particularly open to differing presentations in public and private accounts (Wilson 1987).

In addition to differences in accounts there is also the possibility that actual behaviour will differ from the interview account. An interview does not give very much scope for checking the congruence of accounts and behaviours, but it is sometimes possible to record differences. Stories of real happenings may contradict more general accounts based on acceptable stereotypes. Alternatively the visit may include more than just an interview. For example, a woman who stated, in the context of traditional food habits, that her husband always had meat and two vegetables for his main meal, later displayed a stack of cook-chill meals in the freezer. This case illustrates how meanings and interpretations may differ for researchers and respondents. Alternatively it can be seen as an example of the way that the meaning of public accounts alters so that behaviour in advanced old age can be harmonized with life-long traditional values.

Stereotypical gender relations in advanced old age

Men's roles outside the home

According to popular stereotypes of gender roles, men take paid work and have work-related social lives or hobbies while women rear children and cook, clean and wash. Women are also expected to build and maintain social contacts in the family and away from the workplace. The strength of these gender stereotypes was such that in two couple interviews women described their lives in terms of being at home while the man was out, only to be corrected by the husband, who pointed out that things were different since he had retired 15 to 20 years ago. In these cases the gap between the stereotypical public account and the gendered reality in later life was clearly identified by the men. In other cases it may not have been. The other major discrepancy between stereotype and reality was that virtually all the women had taken paid work at some point in their lives, even if this was only before they married, or during World War II.

In advanced old age the stereotypes of gender relations no longer applied over large areas of daily life. The old roles had gone, but no new ways of behaving had been socially prescribed, possibly because until recently advanced old age has not been a common life stage. Men did not work. Only a handful of men were able to keep up a pattern of going out alone daily for long periods, rarely to business, often to a hobby such as an allotment. Five out of 42 men were still working part time, but with one exception (a 91-year-old organ player), they belonged to the younger members of the sample. For some, the extra income from work was essential to their standard of living (particularly the ability to run a car). A few others liked to go out by themselves. A number had retired at the conventional age from full time work and taken a part time job until around age 75.

Other aspects associated with masculinity, such as work-related social activities, were also largely absent in the sample. Single-sex bowling, ex-servicemen's clubs and Freemasonry were the only reported examples of single-sex social activities for men. Thus very few married men had social lives that did not include their wives. The great majority were no longer able to continue their earlier activities for a range of reasons. Lack of money was a restriction which applied to middle-class as well as working-class men. They could not afford to 'stand rounds' in the club or pub. Physical strength or ill health were other constraints.

The need to withdraw from social life, which Cumming and Henry (1966) saw as a characteristic of old age, was frequently articulated. It was not clear how far men felt that they had to give up activities, or offices that they had held in clubs and societies, because of socially held perceptions that they were 'too old', and how far they acted because they themselves *felt* 'too old', that is, did they withdraw freely or were they pushed? Given an ageist society, the distinction is almost impossible to make objectively, but in terms of personal perceptions it could be important. A few men did have social roles in local horticultural societies and in clubs based outside the area such as local history groups, but in most cases, even if these had been important activities in early retirement, they were reduced or had ceased by the time the men were interviewed.

There appeared to be very few social activities available for men in advanced old age outside their own families. Far fewer men than women were present at virtually all the social activities reported. This was felt to be intimidating or distasteful to many men but did not seem to affect the women. Women were more likely to say that they did not like the company of old *people* while men specifically mentioned not liking the company of old *women*. Some said that they did not take part in local activities because they were 'too feminine'.

In contrast there were men who appeared to do everything with their wives; couples who were inseparable, where each relied wholly on the other and who had little contact with other people. A more frequent pattern was for married men to rely substantially on their wives but not wholly. In most cases this meant that they had access to a wider range of activities outside the home than those who were widowers. The exceptions were four widowers or divorced men who had relationships with women. They reported visits, foreign holidays, trips to visit their friends' relatives and cultural outings which they took part in as a couple.

Men's roles inside the home

Although men were much more likely to maintain gender roles within the home than outside it, even here gender divisions were weakened in advanced old age. One former printer had decided to take over the housework soon after he retired (having formerly employed a cleaner). As he said 'I'm the au pair'. Another husband insisted on cooking for himself, which enabled him to eat when and what he wanted. Men who were widowers of necessity had to take on activities that were stereotypically female. Daughters or daughters-in-law might help, but since in this sample none were co-resident, widowed older men cooked and cleaned. Some husbands with disabled wives also took on fairly heavy loads of cooking, shopping or washing (mostly collecting clothes from the launderette). As one disabled wife said:

Mrs W: But he's a wonderful head cook and bottle washer.
Interviewer: Do you enjoy doing that?
Mr W: Yes, it's no hardship at all.

Shopping was frequently a male activity in later life. One man mentioned the company of meeting other pensioners at the supermarket check-out.

The men in the sample were also less able to continue traditional male tasks within the home than they had been when younger and this led to regrets. As one said:

I used to do everything in the house but now, of course, the house needs repainting. It hurts me to give this sort of job to someone who wouldn't do such a good job as I would do myself, and I would have to pay him.

Some still decorated and repaired but at a very much reduced level. Others had given up entirely for a range of health reasons. Working-class men had formerly cleaned the outside of windows but they were unable to do the upper storeys and many could no longer do the ground floor windows either.

The archetypal male activity for all except the poorest members of the sample had been car driving. (Very few women in this generation had learned to drive.) In advanced old age few men were able to afford to run a car. Those that did either had large savings or still worked part time and were able to finance the car through their earnings. However, most of these men were unable to drive far and as one said, 'the car is only a shopping basket'. Others reported dramatic reductions in their social lives once they stopped driving. One was no longer able to help other pensioners with shopping, lifts and other social activities. Nor was he able to visit his daughter as he had in the past. Another described how he had to give up going to bowls since he was not able to drive after a minor stroke. He did not feel that it would be right to arrive at his bowls club in a taxi. Another widower had seen his hopes of companionship fade when his car failed the MOT and a reduction in his part time earnings meant that he could not afford to repair it. He could no longer drive to visit his 'lady friend' who lived the other side of London. Many recalled the freedom to make visits and go on spontaneous trips which the car had brought in early retirement.

Watching television could be seen as a gendered activity in terms of programme choice but this was very much an area where couples tended to report common tastes, as in 'We don't like a lot of what's on television these days.' It was clear that men watched or listened to more news and sports programmes. Even so, life was relatively limited for the majority of men. As one said, addressing first his wife and then the interviewer:

> You've kept a lot of your friends, more than I have. She used to run the Girl Guides and has always helped with these sort of things. I'm more inclined to sit down and watch football on the television.

Men's other chief domestic role, that of provider and manager of money is heavily class biased. While the men in the sample had higher incomes on average than the women, and nearly all men had bigger pensions than their wives, a few women had full state pensions and a handful had substantial personal incomes. In working-class households, women had traditionally managed the money and as Townsend (1957) pointed out in his study of older people in the 1950s, working-class women were often relatively well off in later life because they got their own state pensions and continued to manage a share of their husband's money. Most middle-class men continued to manage the money until frailty prevented them. At that point their wives had to take over. Wives used words which indicated that they saw themselves, or represented themselves in couple interviews, as less capable with money than their husbands, even though this was no longer true (if it ever had been).

The gendered division of labour was not clear in respect of gardening. The stereotypical division was between men who grew vegetables and women who grew flowers, but this was not adhered to in later life and only one man in the sample still kept up his allotment. As mentioned above nearly all members of the sample were responsible for a garden. It appeared that gardening was an activity where personal choice could be exercised, free of gender stereotyping.

Many men were flower gardeners and always had been. Widowers who had been married to keen gardeners or men whose wives could no longer garden, easily, did not take over this role. However those who enjoyed gardening were able to continue even when in very poor health.

Women's gendered roles

Care of children in succeeding generations was of limited relevance in determining women's roles in advanced old age. Those with children had brought them up and had often made a major contribution to bringing up their grandchildren (who were now nearly all adults), but no one recorded bringing up a third generation of children. This did not mean they had no contact with great-grandchildren but rather that they were not taking responsibility for childcare at the time of the interviews. This finding might have been a specific feature of the sample, rather than of women in advanced old age in general. In more closely knit communities, great-grandmothers may still be doing a significant amount of childcare. Help in emergencies was reported but it was clear that such emergencies had grown rare in recent years, while they had been very common, especially in the working-class area, in the early years of retirement.

Women continued to take most responsibility for domestic work for as long as they were able. However they often reported that their attitudes to it had changed and they did less. Sometimes this was through choice and sometimes because of disability. A few middle-class women had always employed cleaners. Other women felt forced to once they could no longer manage the housework themselves and knew they were ineligible for a home help. Husbands might complain, but they had little choice.

Stereotypical gender roles were different for women who belonged to the relatively large proportion of their cohort who had never married (15 out of 89). Others had had no children – again a cohort experience since birthrates were very low in the interwar depression years. For them the issue of childcare had not arisen, though most had looked after elderly parents or other relatives.

As with the men, paid work was no longer an issue for the women in the sample. Only two were still doing any paid work. Very few married women or widows had had careers in the modern sense of the term. Their paid work had often been intermittent and had been fitted in around caring responsibilities. One single woman had given up her intermittent work in journalism to look after her parents. She was over 40 when both died and she was able to begin professional training. After qualifying she tried to enter politics and continued in professional work until the age of 84 and to campaign until 90. Other women with the same early life pattern of work that was not taken seriously by patriarchal fathers, followed by a long time spent caring, were less able to assert themselves in later life. However only one of the single women had never undertaken paid work.

The women in the sample were in general much more closely involved with their families than men. Most had much wider social lives. A similar finding has been recorded by Matthews (1986), Keith (1989), and Jerrome (1993). Women, even married women, were able to socialize by themselves. They were not restricted to women-only activities. As one husband said: 'She won't have any dirty thoughts at this age, so it doesn't matter if she meets men'. Evening classes, Townswomen's Guild, Pensioner's Link and a range of activities at local clubs were among the activities mentioned by women. Single women also reported visits to friends and to theatres and concerts in much the same way as married women, whereas single men were less likely to do so unless they had a friend of the opposite sex.

Continuity and change as they affect gender relations in advanced old age

Marital status is a key factor in any discussion of gender relations in advanced old age, particularly for men. Continuity was the dominant characteristic of most marital relationships. The stress on continuity may be one reason why it is so important to both men and women to maintain lifelong gender distinctions. For example in one couple the wife had always managed the money and, although nearly blind, she was still firmly in charge of most aspects of the marriage:

W: I do the shopping, but he's watching me all the time.
H: I watch her. Sometimes she mixes up the money, the coins.
W: The coins. I've got two purses and I have to have every coin in a different compartment so I know where they are.
H: And I, I don't dive in to her. I let her carry on because otherwise we'd be embarrassed. So I give her a fair hand, you know, until I have to step in behind her – or not. But um – otherwise we haven't got much to worry about really.

Here the embarrassment that would result if the wife was shown as no longer able to fill her gendered role is the issue, rather than any personal concerns about male power. The general impression was that, in close marriages, issues of power had faded as issues of daily survival became increasingly important (also see Rose and Bruce's Chapter 9).

The quotation in the title of this chapter, 'I'm the eyes and she's the arms', expresses a degree of dependence and role reversal which may be inevitable where one or both partners is severely disabled. In this case the man's heart condition prevented him from doing almost all physical activity and his wife could not see. However such closeness did not necessarily depend on physical disability. Another couple spent every fine afternoon walking round London markets and had almost no social contacts apart from each other. Rawlins reported similar relationships in old age. One man said 'Because we're so close, we're just one. We do everything together' (1992: 267).

These close marriages appeared to be a highly satisfactory way of living later life but they depended on a delicate balance of capabilities in the couple. If one partner became too disabled or died the other was left with very limited social resources. This was particularly true for childless couples or those whose children were distant either geographically or emotionally.

Other less close marriages showed similar patterns in which gendered power divisions were weakened. Women had more freedom to conduct their lives as they wished as long as their health, or the health of their partner, allowed them. Some used ill health as a reason for reducing their performance of gendered tasks (by cutting back on housework or cooking or employing help), but it was not clear from the interviews how far this was a positive choice and how far it was forced upon them.

Single women were also characterized by a high degree of continuity from earlier to later life in most cases. Many had never been very interested in domestic activities and certainly did less as they got older. One women of 94 spoke enthusiastically about her meals on wheels, whereas women who had been used to cooking were much more critical. Another single woman said of food: 'I *can* cook, but by the time you've bought the stuff, you've prepared it, you've cooked it, you put it on the table, its old news and you're bored with it.'

Most of the single women had had well developed networks of friends and relatives which they had built up without the restraints on women's social life that often came from marriage. These networks were shrinking and losses were hard to replace as contemporaries died or went into distant residential homes. Women who had been widowed early shared many of the character-istics of those who had never married. They had been in paid work and usually had relatively good pensions. Like most of the single women, they visited a range of friends and could afford to hire cars when they needed transport – mostly to carry luggage to trains, coach stations or airports.

There was much less continuity for those who were widowed later in life. Widows and widowers had to cope with major change both in gendered roles and relationships and in their images of self. Often they were in poor health and debilitated by a period of caring or coping with insensitive services which did not respond to their needs.

Problems of gender relations in advanced old age

Socially approved models of gender relations are very limited in advanced old age. Writers have noted that new relationships between men and women can attract disapproval from the peer group as well as from younger generations (Hockey and James 1993). Rawlins (1992) found that older people made a point of describing new relationships as highly respectable. Masculinity in later life might be hard to express. One man explained how he had not known how to behave when beginning a friendship with a woman:

> I was in the health centre and a lady said 'What about you getting home?' and she said 'You can use the phone in my house', and I said 'Oh no thank you'. I was frightened, terrified, but anyway I did visit her in the end and where she lives it's like a corner house and the garden is down the back quite a long way and you can see for miles. She said 'Come upstairs and have a look', and I thought what am I going upstairs for into her bedroom. I wasn't being dirty or anything but I was really afraid of her. When I talk about it now I have to laugh about it because it's true, I was frightened. The son is very nice, I get on well with him and I said to him 'I was terrified of your mother, I thought she was trying to get me on the bed to rape me but as old as I am I was terrified of her'. To meet someone like that after 50 or 60 years, you don't know how to act. You don't know what to do or say. And the first time I went there strange to say, I just gave her a peck on the cheek. She didn't like it. She didn't think it was right. So we both were embarrassed about one another.

The relationship had worked well despite extreme frailty on both sides. It had also been accepted by both sets of children.

The women in the sample who had formed new relationships with men showed no desire to marry. This contrasted with widowed men who were much more likely to want to marry. As one man said of his second marriage: 'We married for company and that, and it's worked very well.' Women were less likely to see marriage as a way of getting company. In their relationships with male friends they exchanged services, such as cooking and mending, for gardening and do-it-yourself and went on trips together. The difference from marriage lay in the power relationships involved. As unmarried friends, women were more able to choose what to do and when. Companionship was appreciated by both men and women but their aims in later life were not symmetrical. Laslett (1989a: 137) notes that historically widows who had some standing were less likely to marry again.

Constraints on a redefinition of gender identities

Women, in general, had more choices in gender roles and in ways of expressing gendered identities in advanced old age, while men had fewer. Both, however, faced constraints on their activities if they wished to change their gendered roles in any way (and of course many, possibly the majority, of the sample did not). For those who were frail or in poor health the main aim, as they often expressed it, was 'just to keep going from day to day', something which took very large amounts of time and energy. In these circumstances change is not usually undertaken in later life unless it is forced by ill health or some catastrophe. For example, a woman disabled by a car crash was forced to give up housework and her husband had to try and take over. Neither viewed the change as positive.

Another constraint on their freedom, and for many of the sample the most important, was the family. Widows and widowers who had the chance to alter the way they lived when no longer constrained by a partner often found that any attempt at change was stopped or criticized by their families. Children were recorded as disapproving of new relationships or constantly requesting parents not to take the risks involved in travelling to visit friends or going on holiday. Women were requested not to do their own housework or not to become vegetarian. Children were reported as being generally controlling and anti-change.

Other lifelong or society-wide gendered constraints existed or were exacerbated by old age. Some recently widowed women still reported finding it hard to socialize without a man. There was widespread fear of crime and of going out alone after dark even in the better-off neighbourhood. This fear was most often reported by women but it had spread to some men. Outside contacts and activities were limited by mobility and the problems generated by inadequate public transport – stairs, late trains, and buses that were impossible to get on or off when carrying shopping.

Age, cohort or secular trend?

This study showed clear indications of an *age affect*. In advanced old age both men and women, but particularly men, appeared to be less concerned with the power aspects of gender relations than they had been in the past. The emphasis on survival and just keeping going did not leave much room for gender-based assertions of domestic power and there were virtually no power-based roles outside the household available to men in advanced old age. Men appeared to have mellowed in their old age. Married women were sometimes able to benefit from this decline in the power of men to redefine gender in old age. Many were able to have a freer social life, to do more things they enjoyed and less housework, especially cooking.

The positive effects of ageing in terms of gender relations were balanced by the negative effects of reduced physical capabilities. Ill health was one serious and limiting problem for some of the sample. Those who were not obviously ill still found that most things took longer to do and so they could do less. Some things that they had done in the past were beyond their current capacity. Other negative effects of ageing were related to diminishing social networks. Longer life meant greater chances of loss of friends and relatives through institutionalization and death.

Cohort effects were also clearly evident. The number of single women was abnormally high in the cohorts studied, in comparison with those before and after them. Single women had entered the labour market and enjoyed greater opportunities for independence and the development of new forms of gender relations than married women of the same birth cohort. They provided a comparator group because they differed from the more stereotypically conventional life course of the other women in their cohort. It could be argued that, by following an alternative lifestyle, they helped to develop a more favourable climate for changing gender relations for all women in their cohort. Cohort effects could also be seen in the way that respondents recalled the inter-war depression years. Their experience of hardship when young was seen as helpful in coping with the privations of old age.

Period (or secular) changes had clearly helped to improve the position of women as far as the sample was concerned. Both men and women agreed that the division of labour had been very much more marked in the past. The picture presented was one in which men went out to work (unless they were unemployed in the interwar years) and did nothing about the house when they returned. Women, on the other hand, did a great deal of heavy housework and in many families took paid work as well. Gender roles were not only identified as having been clearer in the past, but were also seen as more inequitable.

The other major secular change which had affected this sample was the reduction in poverty for the working class and the increase in prosperity for the middle class. This, combined with their experience of the interwar years, gave most members of the sample a feeling that they were better off than they had expected and that they could cope with privation thanks to their past experiences.

Conclusions

Some of the observations noted above are specific to the two cohorts studied. In future there will be very few women who have never married, but the place of single women will be taken by divorcées who are likely to share some of the characteristics of single women, depending on how long they have lived alone. Like the single women in the sample, they are likely to develop new ways of expressing gendered identities in advanced old age.

The rate of change in gender relations in advanced old age may be reduced if the average life expectancies of men and women become more similar and women's period of widowhood is reduced. The interviews showed that marriage was a site of control of women by men, even in advanced old age, so longer marriage may reinforce conventional gender relations. However, the study also showed that even within marriage, women in advanced old age were able to reduce many of the more burdensome aspects of the gendered division of labour and to achieve greater freedom in terms of their social lives.

As a greater proportion of people reach advanced old age, it is possible that a socially approved life stage may develop which older people can accept as their own, rather than having to construct their lives without any positive models. Women's values would be likely to be more dominant than they are at earlier ages, if only because their numbers would be greater. However, new socially approved ways of living in advanced old age have to compete with a postmodern approach to the life course which sees each individual as engaged in their own life project (see Chapter 2). Gender identities and gender relations which are positive and satisfying for women are less likely to develop if life becomes a 'reflexive project' with individuals working out their own identities, rather than forming a 'defined collectivity' Giddens (1991: 33). The individual approach demands material resources which the majority of women in later life are unlikely to have. It is easier for the majority of women to conform to a new collectivity than to engage in reflexive projects which develop individual autonomous ways of living.

At present it can be argued that ageing into advanced old age allows a reworking or re-evaluation of gender roles in a range of different directions. Couples may find that togetherness becomes the main aspect of their lives: 'intimacy beyond the dreams of youth' (Friedan 1993). Alternatively they may live close, but separate, lives with greater freedom for women to do as they wish and a narrowing of gender roles for men who are no longer in paid work and often do not have the strength to perform traditional male household tasks. In either case stereotypical gender roles are altered and reduced.

It is still unclear how the changes noted above relate to age, cohort and period effects. Age is clearly very important, but period, in terms of the feminist movement and the improved economic position of women, also has a major effect. The respondents themselves identified cohort effects, in terms of their experience of hardship in their early years, as one of the central influences on their perception of their current lifestyles as generally satisfactory.

Acknowledgements

I am indebted to the Nuffield Foundation for financing the research on which this chapter is based and to Tami Desai for assistance with computer-aided qualitative data analysis.

9

MUTUAL CARE BUT DIFFERENTIAL ESTEEM: CARING BETWEEN OLDER COUPLES

Hilary Rose and Errollyn Bruce

The debate about the gender division of informal caring stemmed from the pioneering feminist research of the 1970s and early 1980s which conceptualized caring as an integral aspect of the domestic labour debate. Despite the collapse of the domestic labour debate it had reclaimed both housework and caring as reproductive work and thus as integral to the social division of labour. As a labour process, caring was characterized as a mix of both hard physical and complex emotional work. The feminist literature distinguished between caring for and caring about (Ungerson 1987), while the mainstream social policy literature less satisfactorily distinguished between tending and caring (Parker 1981). This early feminist research sought to bring women's lives to the foreground in order to give them both theoretical and political value. However it was left to non-academic older feminists such as Mary Stott to offer a non-pathologizing approach to both age and gender. Her *Ageing for Beginners* (1981) was part of a social and intellectual movement against the pathologizing of ageing, taken up later by feminist sociologists (e.g. Arber and Ginn 1991a; Bernard and Meade 1993).

The sociology of caring debate, like feminism itself, is international, but national context produces difference; thus British research reflected the interests of the dominant generation and ethnicity of the women's movement, with the result that the initial research was almost exclusively concerned with the problems of white younger and middle-aged women (Finch and Groves 1980, 1983). Thus in the edited collection *Women and the Life Cycle* (Allatt *et al.* 1987), only Mason (1987) considered women of pensionable age and even Oakley's (1987) discussion of gender and generation implicitly equates the menopause with the outer limit of generation. Even where informal care was provided by neighbours it was predominantly provided by women (Abrams *et al.* 1989). The thesis that women were the universal informal carers became part of a feminist political culture. It was for example, taken up and both reflected and constituted by the Equal Opportunities Commission (1980, 1982), disseminated widely through the many local authority women's committees of the 1980s and was widely researched and taught in Women's Studies and Social Policy courses. It was valuable in that it provided a more sharply focused criticism of 'community care', that favourite of a patriarchal left and right alike, as the means whereby governments and social service departments transferred a public and collective responsibility on to individuals, mainly women.

However there was a high theoretical and political price of attributing agency only to this single valorized group, leaving elderly people – both women and men – to be conceptualized as passive objects (Finch and Groves 1980, 1983; Walker 1982; Ungerson 1983, 1987; Marsden and Abrams 1987; Henderson 1988; Lewis and Meredith 1988; Finch and Mason 1993), and erased, along with those outside the dominant culture. The criticism from the disability movement (Begum 1991), from older feminists (Stacey 1989), from carers (Briggs and Oliver 1985), and from black feminism (Carby 1982) charged that a feminism, unaware of its own 'race', able bodiedness and age, had in its desire to cease to be the Other constructed Other Others. By the 1980s white men too began to complain, as part of a general restiveness within cultural politics, that those men who did care were also being erased (Bytheway 1987; Fisher 1993). This complaint received some support from feminist sociologists who saw the concept of gender as central to the discussion of ageing (Arber and Gilbert 1989a; Arber and Ginn 1991a). Such shifts within the caring debates echoed the larger canvas covered by the Women's Studies–Men's Studies–Gender Studies debates. By the 1990s a very much more complex account of caring, gender and ageing had emerged, which recognized that it ought to pay attention to differences of ethnicity and 'race'.

By contrast, Scandinavian research, set in the context of the friendly state (not a concept available to British feminists), focused on relational aspects of caring. Ve (1984), in an important early paper, distinguished between three forms of informal care: mutual care as between equals such as friends, necessary care for survival such as care of the very young or very sick or very old, and personal servicing which was extracted by patriarchal power by ablebodied men from women. This influential account created political space to endorse certain forms of informal caring while resisting others. Thus in this chapter we use the concept of mutual care for the equal exchange of the caring relationship of some older couples at a particular stage of their lives. The Scandinavian perspective also fostered approaches which conceptualized paid carers not as agents of social control (Wilson 1975) – the dominant UK perspective – but as solidaristic towards the cared for (Eliasson 1989; Simonen 1990). The British equal opportunities approach projected a negative experience of personal service care on to all forms of care but especially those involving the care of mothers by daughters. The construction of care in the Scandinavian literature, which involved a conception of the rights of the cared for along with those of the carers, was not visible within the collectively undersupported British climate.

Caring in the context of a withering welfare state

Since the Conservative government came to power in 1979, the debates around community care took place in a context of an increasingly fierce attack on the principle of collective welfare and of increasing moves by elderly people with resources to seek new solutions. For older people and their carers this diminished commitment was marked by the official report *Growing Older* (DHSS 1981) which, echoing the parallel German discussion of subsidiarity as the crucial principle within welfare, emphasized that the:

> primary sources of support and care for elderly people are informal and voluntary. These spring from personal ties of kinship, friendship and neighbourhood. They are irreplaceable. It is the role of public authorities to sustain and where necessary develop – but never displace – such support and care. Care in the community must increasingly mean care by the community.
>
> (DHSS 1981: 1)

In this context the response of carers' organizations was to stress the commonalities of caring and campaign for more practical help, such as respite care and more flexible domiciliary services. Feminism's more utopian thinking stressed collective solutions (Dalley 1988) or looked to men to share more of the caring so as to construct a more altruistic society (Land and Rose 1985). The grass roots organizations, on the other hand, campaigned for concrete and immediate gains which would support the carers and the cared for. Inspection of these apparently rival proposals indicates that they are not in fundamental competition with one another but rather reflect the multiplicity of levels which need addressing.

Once universalism ceased to have a strong political grip on social policy formation, issues of the political leverage of generations markedly influenced the extent to which governments felt the need to counter critical research. Unlike the young homeless, the older generation commands a considerable segment of the vote and is less easily abandoned. Thus even though most of the pioneering feminist research was based on small samples, typically recruited from health and welfare agencies, the findings were sufficiently politically potent (not least because of the pressure from a pervasive feminist movement) to stimulate the governmental General Household Survey (GHS) to explore the same issues in a large scale survey (Green 1988).

The 1985 GHS findings that older male spouses did almost as much caring as older female spouses were received with considerable suspicion in feminist circles. It was widely argued that a number of the tabulations in the 1985 GHS survey artefactually created an equality of caring tasks – for example, that keeping an eye on an elderly neighbour or helping out with transport (which as Wenger, 1984, observes are common forms of support and care given by men in a rural context) is treated as the equivalent of changing soiled sheets. The GHS asked about 'extra family responsibilities' which assumes that everyone knows what 'normal' family responsibilities are, thus inviting underreporting by women against a bureaucratically determined normalcy (Green 1988, 1990).

Getting older in Nortown

Since only a tiny minority of older people are admitted to institutional care, it follows that where the material circumstances make it both possible and necessary, and partners share an ideology of love and duty (perhaps less romantically conceptualized as independence and commitment to being in a couple), then gendered constructions of caring must give way to the pragmatics of coping. It was this we decided to explore empirically in a study of older couples in Nortown. A considerable body of evidence, such as that brought together by Arber and Ginn (1991a), suggests that where both partners are still at home the extreme dependency which may occur with physiological ageing is likely to be accepted pragmatically as a natural extension of co-residence and long relationship, and that the gender divisions of care which had operated earlier in the life course would hold less rigidly. Despite this probable change in conventional gender division of tasks, would the experience and performance of care itself be gendered? Thus our focus was on the relational aspects – what was the interplay of ageing, changing and deepening dependency and gender? And how did these operate in a multicultural context?

   To explore these questions we selected a random sample of 1000 men and 1000 women over 65 drawn from the age-sex register of a general practice in Nortown, a small highly multicultural northern city (Bruce and Rose 1994). Postal questionnaires were sent out, and 989 were returned enabling us to identify couples where one partner was heavily dependent and the other was the main carer. Identifying carers was based on the tasks which they reported doing for their partner, their sense of looking after them, and the reported level of disability of their partner. From these couples where there was a clear carer and cared for, we drew a subsample of 16 couples, eight where the man was more dependent and eight where the woman was more dependent. We used simultaneous but separate interviewing to give the interviewees space for some self-representation as autonomous beings, and to speak of matters that they might not wish to share with their partner (Townsend 1957; Edwards 1980; Pahl 1989).

The postal questionnaire was successful in identifying carers but proved too coarse an instrument for exploring the details of the labour process, especially the distribution of emotional labour. Only the more open approach of an interview allowed people to describe how the experience of caring is shaped as much by what it means to be doing certain tasks, as by the actual doing of them.

Slippery facts and the labour process

We wanted to explore in detail the kind of caring tasks and household chores carried out by the carers and the cared for, conscious that women and men feel very differently about these tasks (Ungerson 1983). Like Arber and Gilbert (1989b) we found that mutual care frequently preceded the situation in which the dichotomy between the carer and the cared for became evident. Thus we were interested to ask how the gender division of tasks had changed over time, as well as to explore what tasks were currently done, especially those that were done reluctantly.

Some carers were keen to communicate the full details of a situation that they experienced as distressingly abnormal, whereas others minimized their accounts of the help they gave, out of loyalty to their partner and a joint desire to present everything as more or less normal to the outside world. This effect was illustrated by how the carer reported the cared for partner's contribution to the household. For example a person with dementia who was able to peel the potatoes when given equipment and instructions could be reported as helping with domestic tasks; however, the carer might not experience this as help at all, since it takes far more time and energy to organize and supervise the task than to perform it. The same action, in this case potato peeling, could be seen as a small but valuable contribution to the domestic workload or as yet another responsibility for the carer, namely, providing and supervising an appropriate activity. Similarly potting out seedlings on the kitchen table by a paraplegic man required a substantial amount of preparation and clearing up by his partner – thus was simultaneously both a contribution by him to household tasks and a further burden on her.

The alternative ways in which caring tasks may be experienced and reported was exemplified by a physically highly dependent woman, Mrs Anderson – (fictional names are used in the chapter), who was unable to be on her own, but frequently had her small grandchildren to visit. While explaining that she and her husband could only cope with one grandchild at a time it was very clear that she saw herself, despite her physical infirmity, as personally controlling and taking emotional care of her grandchildren. She needed them to be physically self-sufficient but gained great satisfaction in contributing to their emotional well-being, not least because their father had died and she felt they needed extra support. Invisible emotional work such as this was not seen as work but part of family life. Even more so, emotional labour on one's own feelings was a large part of the invisible work carried out by carer and cared for as they struggled to survive disabilities and illnesses which were laying siege to their quality of life (James 1989). What had at first seemed simple matters of fact had a slippery coating of feelings and meanings. By putting together the accounts from both partners we were able to observe not simply how tasks had, in some cases, been over or underreported on the postal questionnaire but also what had been conceptualized as a task and what was taken as natural to being a gendered partner, parent and grandparent.

Necessity and negotiation

With many tasks, carers felt that they had no choice, given the circumstances, but to perform them. For the cared for, the inability to do things which they had done in the past, either for the couple or for themselves, was a matter of continuing regret and for some of them, rage. Mrs Anderson, who had always looked after their joint money but whose eyesight now failed her, and who could neither put on her makeup nor do her hair, spoke of retreating to the privacy of the toilet to weep at her lost capacities. Nonetheless, feeling able to complain about the quality of life, to speak of days where the only self-description was 'I'm a bloody mess today', was only possible for those with a strong emotional as well as practical support structure. For Mrs Anderson, this was the presence of a loving if controlling husband, a close daughter and loving grandchildren.

Both carer and cared for acknowledged bodily imperatives in all their untidy urgency. If someone needs the toilet, and cannot manage alone, whoever happens to be in the house at that moment must assist, regardless of gender preferences. Coping was often achieved through pragmatic denial: 'I just blank my mind'. Nonetheless, there were strong feelings about violating cross-gender taboos (Ungerson 1983, 1987), so where needs were less pressing, ways could be found to avoid certain tasks. A common example is personal washing. Several men had organized daughters to come in to give their mothers a weekly bath, but they coped with the daily personal wash themselves. Intergenerational same gender care was mostly seen by men as preferable to cross-gender care between spouses.

Denial was also a means of coping when the situation made this practicable. One woman described how she gave her handicapped husband an all over wash, but left him with a bowl of water to wash 'down there', saying that she didn't really know how well he managed. Other women remained in the room while bathing their husbands, but handed them a pre-soaped flannel and instructed them to do their own 'twiddly bits'.

However, where incontinence makes washing intimate parts of the body essential at unpredictable times of day and night, qualms about the job have to be set aside; the remaining choice is separation, loneliness for the carer and institutionalization of the cared for. However, before this extreme point of dependency has been reached, the solutions to the problem of personal care

120   HILARY ROSE AND ERROLLYN BRUCE

are enormously varied. They result from a process of negotiation around what has to be done, what each partner finds tolerable or intolerable, and their perceptions of the sources of help available to them. Carers described how they talked themselves and their partners into doing and accepting such services. Comforting commonplace expressions, which both understated the severity of the challenge and simultaneously acknowledged changes in bodily capacities over the years, were used to make the hitherto taboo behaviour acceptable. As Gail Wilson (Chapter 8) documents, length of shared life serves to soften the negotiation.

Evidence from the mutual carers identified in the postal questionnaire suggests that flexibility over gender divisions of tasks is understood as necessary to maintain highly-valued independence as a couple. For these couples, what was of paramount importance was to manage jointly without help from beyond the household, to maintain reciprocal relationships with their children, and to avoid bringing in outsiders to do tasks which they had previously managed themselves. As one elderly husband wrote: 'Surely all men over 80 help in the house, if only a little'. A woman commented: 'We both do what we can and both look after one another as best we can', capturing the sense of satisfaction in coupledom so striking in this group, but also acknowledging that physiological ageing can bring limitations.

None of these mutual carers were facing the extremes of dependency typical of the couples interviewed; however, periods of illness and minor disabilities made dependency a salient issue for them, and they give a forceful illustration of the ideology which is so impossible for the care couples to live up to, but which influences their negotiation of solutions to dependency. Thus the over-riding desire for independence as a couple erodes previously gender-determined allocations of tasks, even before the demands of extreme depen-dency leave little choice other than to do what needs doing or to accept separation and institutionalization.

Although these negotiations are reported here as if they were between individuals they are contextualized by the lack of availability of state support in terms of provision and care from social service departments. They are very conscious of the inadequacy of state support. These couples may have a modest economic sufficiency or near sufficiency, but many are anxious about bills, especially fuel bills.

The underrepresentation of women in very heavy caring situations

As the interviewing proceeded we found fewer women than men in very 'heavy' caring situations and suspected a bias in the selection of the interviews. A phone survey of the uninterviewed eligible couples showed among the 'unwilling to be interviewed' a striking difference between the reasons given by women and by men carers. Apart from three rather reclusive respondents, both genders were very willing to talk on the telephone about their circumstances and give their reasons. The men carers were not in particularly demanding caring situations; their reasons for not wishing to be interviewed related to mild inconvenience. In contrast seven of the eight women carers were in very demanding situations, four of them had refused interviews because their husbands would not have liked it, although they often talked at some length on the phone. In all these cases the husbands were resistant to help from strangers, preferring help from family members. One man did not like social calls from anyone except the family, while another refused to let his wife take a break. These are very small numbers, but suggest that wives in heavy caring situations are less likely to agree to an interview than men carers, because they are anxious to avoid upsetting either precarious routines or difficult men. There was a grimly familiar tone to the conversations with these women who felt unable to invite us to their homes because of their husbands' dislike of outsiders and visitors, which resonated with the many accounts in the feminist literature of the ways in which women's lives can be controlled by the demands of men.

There was also evidence from the interviews that there were times when men's preferences and predilections – whether as carers or cared for – had greater weight in the process of negotiation than women's. One woman with multiple sclerosis did not like being left on her own in the house while her husband went out for a daily walk, but said that she knew that he needed it. Another did not really like her husband washing her intimately, and was conscious that it was his views, not hers, which prevented her from going to day care. Several men but no women carers arranged interviews without consulting their partners, in one case despite the fact that the wife (who had Alzheimer's disease) disliked strangers and was inclined to get agitated and violent when upset. Where there are long histories of greater consideration given to men's needs this pattern is likely to persist, and to be so 'normal' to the spouses that it is either not noticed at all or too obvious to mention.

Whereas both male and female carers expressed their inability to enjoy themselves while out, for fear of what might be happening at home, none of our male carers expressed the feeling that they must compensate for their wives' suffering. Wives seemed to be striving to compensate for their husband's losses in various ways, sometimes by depriving themselves, as in the following example of an older woman who looked after her husband with dementia. Although he showed signs of insecurity when left with a sitter while she went out, and it made no difference to him what she did while she was away, she nevertheless said: 'You see my daughters said to me. "Have a meal out when that carer comes". But I just can't, I feel when I come back, I feel as if I've robbed him of something.' The feeling that it is indecent to enjoy things in life that one's partner is no longer capable of enjoying was not expressed by men carers, but was common among women carers. We do not mean to underestimate the experiences – common to both male and female carers – of losing previously valued activities and finding it hard to enjoy the breaks they take, but merely to point out that it is women who are particularly vulnerable to denying themselves small pleasures because their husband is incapable of enjoying them as well.

Another inequality of power in caring concerns physical violence. Men caring for wives who become violent due to the effects that dementia or strokes can have on personality appear unthreatened by their wives' physical violence, while women are more likely to express fear. This rests both on a rational appraisal of the actual risks (women on the whole being less strong than men) and on matters of biography (men generally feeling more streetwise and able to use their physical strength to resist violence). This difference in responses to violence led to women carers actively avoiding situations which might upset their partners, fearing bad reactions. Men carers were more likely to do as they pleased, and deal pragmatically with any ensuing negative reactions from their wives.

As with all negotiations, the relative power of the protagonists is a crucial factor in the importance given to their needs. Although sickness and disability are profoundly disempowering, cared for people may have ways to exert power over their carers; old patterns of family power may remain intact, despite declining mental or physical powers. As one woman put it: 'He always did have us running round him, actually', although another took evident satisfaction that her previously violent husband was now physically dependent on her.

Ageing, ethnicity and racism

Three couples from Nortown's minority communities were interviewed; all three were exceptional in that the households had greater access than usual to cultural if not financial capital. The two Asian households had responded to our original questionnaire out of a strong sense of their duty as citizens, and perhaps also out of pride in their handling of a difficult situation. The other couple was Estonian. All three had been able to take advantage of the relatively cheap housing in Nortown which has enabled some people to recreate ethnic and national communities. Thus the Estonian carer explained that when he needed to go out, a neighbour and friend, who came from the same Baltic village where he grew up, sat with his disabled wife. Two other men whom he had known since childhood lived within five minutes' walk of his house.

In one Asian family, the older Singhs co-resided, according to custom, with their eldest son, and personal care for his stroke-disabled mother was provided by his wife and daughter. However, even here gender divisions of tasks were eroded by necessity. During the day, when the women of the house were out at work and school, the husband of the disabled woman would both feed her and take her to the toilet. Two brothers lived a few streets away and if the caring family needed to go away, members of their households would look after the older couple. In the case of longer absences, the elderly couple would go to stay with one of their daughters who lived in nearby towns. The grandfather was very conscious that the care and support with which he was surrounded would be unlikely to exist for his children. He acknowledged the modernity of his grandchildren with pride, but also with loss, for it was how they would live their lives that would mark the change. However, this account of strong internal family support was cross-cut by incidental anecdotes of racism, particularly concerning discrimination in employment.

Response to the postal survey from the large Asian community in Nortown, despite the Urdu on the cover page and the offer of interpreters, was very poor. Our estimate of the response rate, based on identifying ethnicity from surnames, was 16 per cent compared with an overall 60 per cent. A one-page bilingual questionnaire sent out to non-respondents with Asian surnames yielded a 29 per cent response, and confirmed our suspicions that the age and sex register was particularly inaccurate in respect of Asian elders, since nearly a third of the forms returned were from households where there was no resident over 65. Responses indicated considerable diversity in the living situations of older people, with Asian elders living in one, two and three generation households (Bhalla and Blakemore 1981; Gunaratnam 1993). Not all two or three generation households were following the traditional model in which parents co-reside with their eldest son. Mr Singh, although relying on his son to manage the household, still saw himself as head of the family. Some elders were living in isolation, or with one adult child who bore the brunt of the caring responsibilities in a similar manner to the majority community, but with the added problem of finding that services were hard to access or inappropriate to their needs (Mirza 1991). From a fieldwork perspective, social research on gender and ageing which takes racism seriously remains to be done.

Loss and suffering and the discourse of social science

During the field work, we became conscious that the strength of the 'work model' of care has led to insufficient attention to the language of caring and loss employed by the subjects themselves. This goes beyond Ungerson's (1987) accepted point that men tend to speak about caring using the metaphors of their previous occupation. It raises a concern that the public discourse of social science has frequently been unable to conceptualize the private and intense world of suffering and the emotional labour required to make sense of it and manage it. While this is beginning to change, the concept of care as it has been developed within social research, while rescuing care as practical and emotional labour from the private domain, has been much slower to acknowledge and rescue the emotional labour of the cared for.

The concept of care as work is now more or less consensually constructed by carers' organizations, feminist social research and social services but is often still resisted by the carers and the cared for. Caring is still constantly reclaimed by spouse carers as natural, 'it' is what a wife or husband does. While the research on family obligation teases this process apart, the level and management of suffering by the cared for has been excluded in order to bring responsibility and obligation as understood by potential or actual carers into visibility.

Enduring suffering and continuous caring, which was the case for almost all our interviewees, requires a steady rhetorical invocation of those adages and commonplace expressions which enable people to cope whether as carers or as cared for. What makes it possible for an elderly man to get up half a dozen times in the night to see his wife to the bathroom because 'she's a bit rocky on her feet' (she has early Alzheimer's) is to understand how the careful verbal playing down of both her and his problem renders their joint situation manageable. Commonplace expressions both mask and give meaning to caring – 'if the shoe was on the other foot'; 'in sickness and in health'; 'there's no one else'; 'I put one foot in front of the other'; 'you have to laugh'; 'mustn't grumble'; 'there's always someone worse off' – scatter our transcripts. A rhetoric of coping, by rendering situations of unbelievable difficulty manageable, is not one dimensional; it is balanced by a judicious recitation of loss.

Loss has to be managed particularly carefully in front of the partner, when it is their dependency which causes the loss for the speaker. The second marriage of the Jacksons, who had looked forward to an active retirement, had been suddenly cut short by his paralysis. The pleasure in a late second marriage had been marred when her financial uncertainty and difficult relations with his children were no longer offset by shared excursions and activities. Even in very longstanding relationships, the nature of the partner's loss may be very differently constructed by each. Loss, mostly of personal or shared activities no longer possible, of no more holidays or cuddles, or of sex 10 years ago, was common; but loss of relatives now dead, of friends who no longer visit, of not being able to do things for grandchildren, also threads the accounts.

There are strong conversational rules to be followed, in order to tell the story without either the teller or the hearer being overwhelmed. In the event of a threatened breach, where the story-teller is about to be overwhelmed and incapable of continuing, it is necessary for the interviewer to help steer the conversation back, drawing on reassuring commonplaces. The Jacksons had begun by presenting the happy marriage story – but when interviewed alone, Mrs Jackson almost broke down as she reflected on both the quality of her current life and her future. She had never envisaged such a sudden and permanent loss of quality of life.

Loss and commonplace expressions of coping were the weft and warp of both language and the fabric of everyday life for these older people. The length of the relationships had given them time to hone their skills, and those in more recent relationships found it harder. Our interviewees were experienced communicators, enabling us to take part in the interviews, but not infrequently we found tears in our eyes as we listened afterwards to the tapes.

Without the presence of teller and the 'rules' of the communication exchange about loss, we were freer to react to the pain and courage of the accounts.

Gender and community care

One topic of debate in recent years has been whether men carers are offered more help from formal services. After the robust initial claims of gender bias the evidence currently in view is contradictory, and not easy to assess for a number of reasons. Data have mainly come from samples of people known to service providers, therefore excluding the most service-resistant and service-denied people. Services are sparse and support is meagre for all carers; most supporting services go to people who live alone. Factors like the degree of disability of the person cared for, and the age and health status of the person providing care, all affect what happens. Nonetheless as Wenger (1984) stressed, the bulk of the heavy nursing and terminal care of elderly frail people is provided, not by formal care, but by informal care from their partners.

The implementation of the Community Care Act in 1993 has resulted in mainstream social services effort being directed towards more effective management of too few resources. Our interviewees (whom we spoke to just before the new system was implemented) described proposed changes which involved cutting down on direct practical help, typically reducing cleaning help and instead offering shopping help. For service receivers this was seen as an inadequate substitute since cleaning was seen as irreplaceable, while getting shopping organized was often easier and it was perhaps already done by a neighbour or a relative. The ostensible increase in managerial rationality was viewed by recipients, particularly women, as reducing their quality of life, in terms of living in a house where the carpet in a continuously lived-in sitting room was to be now only vacuumed once a fortnight. A key issue is whether the implementation of the new Community Care legislation has resulted in a diminished quality of everyday life. Some of these losses of services are experienced with particular pain by women for it is they who have taken pride in keeping a gleaming house.

Caring men

An important theme, particularly explored in the more psychological literature, has been the gendering of both coping and caring. This has ranged between noting gender difference to suggesting gender superiority largely on the grounds of men's lesser connection. Thus Wenger (1984) has suggested that men experience different problems in caring to women, being more inclined to make heavy weather of the things they are not used to doing, such as domestic tasks. Hicks (1988) argues that men do much better than women in 'coping' in general. Zarit *et al.* (1986) reverse the connectedness arguments of

Gilligan (1982) to suggest that because men are more detached about the person they care for, they are able to cope better. Bury and Holme's (1991) study of people aged over 90 similarly shows that men do rather better. One of the more disturbing findings is from Fitting *et al.* (1986), who gave a battery of tests to 28 men and 26 women caring for their spouse with dementia; a quarter of the men reported that their relationship with the spouse had improved since the onset of dementia.

Reading such analyses of 'coping better but caring less' through the prism of feminist discussions of caring is like looking through the other end of a telescope. The feminist caring literature is multidimensional: from the US, Gilligan (1982), Ruddick (1982, 1989) and Noddings (1984) make arguments about emotional connectedness and moral reasoning; others seek to reconceptualize an abstract masculine rationality as a feminist responsible rationality (Waerness 1987; Rose 1983, 1994); Hochschild (1983) pioneered the discussion of emotional labour and a responsible rationality, and political theorists have suggested that citizenship needs to be retheorized so as to require caring as a civic duty (Jones 1990). Not caring and thus coping better – even doing a better job for the cared for – is tremendously threatening to any part of this feminist agenda. Consequently this chapter will seek to disentangle those issues associated with 'caring less and coping better'.

Perhaps men can gain satisfaction from the bodily presence of their wives, and their own ability to act as protectors and rescuers is enhanced when their wives' dependency is at its greatest. We found some indication of this theme in the men's interviews; as carers they tended to be less distressed by the condition of their partners. Some had developed rather brilliant strategies for producing caring activities which served to diminish the strain on themselves. One creatively reproduced the past, taking his wife who now had Alzheimer's for a car drive, just as he had before she was ill. The drive, getting out of the house, and her peacefulness were refreshing certainly for him and perhaps for her. He also took his wife to the hairdresser's every week for her shampoo and set, relying on a long and continuous relationship with the hairdresser for it to work, and it did. The hairdresser called him 10 minutes before his wife came out from under the drier so that he could be there when she was ready. Even the cared for men (obviously constrained by their condition) tended to stay in control. Mr Jackson, whose wife became so distressed, was, despite being paraplegic, remarkably tranquil about the future. He saw himself as financially quite secure and socially well integrated into the little cul-de-sac where they lived. He had planned that if his wife died before him (she had a poor heart) that he would pay a friend of hers, a neighbour who visited regularly, to take care of him. He seemed confident that he could make this work out should the need arise.

In contrast, rather than taking pleasure in such accomplishments of competently caring for their 'only partially present' partner, the women grieved for lost persons and for a diminished relationship; they did not take such comfort in the accomplishment of care. Caring was what was expected of them and only failure to care brought attention. While respecting the very real suffering of these men and their dedicated caring, we began to think of men's caring as a pet rabbit relationship. A pet rabbit's survival requires conscientious care; indeed its condition is a source of pride for its carer, and the well cared for pet, or rather its owner, receives much admiration. For women, the husband with Alzheimer's fails to become an equivalent pet, so they grieved. Their equally conscientious care – which gave them little or no respite – produced little of the real, if subdued, sense of pride that the men displayed.

Harsh as the pet rabbit metaphor is, it developed through our need to understand what was acting on us as the interviews progressed. Why did we say to one another, particularly as we drove home from interviews, 'What a wonderful man'? Given that we understood ourselves as feminists who were on the lookout for ways in which the construction of masculinity could bring advantages, or inexperience bring difficulty to caring, this endorsement of men gave cause for some considerable wryness. Many older spouse carers and their partners are frequently in awful situations. It was easy, at least while listening to the stories, to become recruited into their accounts; nonetheless there was not the same tendency to name women who were caring as 'wonderful', but then the women portrayed themselves as coping women not as heroines. Reproducing Mr Wonderful was all too easy, but to reproduce such an undifferentiated and stereotypically positive picture of the women carers was not, for we had not been given such an account. Instead women had offered us a less positive, more nuanced, account of the diversity among women, for whom care giving was nonetheless an expected activity. Class differences between the women subjects and ourselves as interviewers obtruded less than in some cross-gender interviews, though we would not accept that sharing the same gender dissolves other differences in research interviews or elsewhere in social life. We took part in a process in which women subjects more easily reveal their feelings and we as women interviewers felt more able to pick these up. Ungerson (1987) reports the difference she experienced between her gender and that of her subjects, particularly how she feels the women say less because they think that she knows more. Part of that tacit knowledge concerns the status of the always gendered speakers.

And yet, all the interviewees delivered their stories in a matter of fact way, designed to save the feelings of the listener. Talking about illness and suffering is understood as socially dangerous. Even so, caring is seen as normal and natural to women, but something special when performed by men. The superior gender brings esteem to a task undervalued when done by women – particularly old women (Itzin 1990a; Arber and Ginn 1991a). One man told us that his neighbours said: 'Really it's a woman's job, what you're doing', and a woman spoke of her husband's Yorkshire pudding: 'it's as good as a woman's'. No one ever spoke of a caring task being manly; at best caring was gender neutral, otherwise regardless of which gender did the work it remained feminine. Like women, men expressed feelings of sadness and resignation, frustration and anger. They were saddened by what had happened to their wives and to their lives. Their advantage seemed to be that merely to attempt to care is admirable in a man, whereas for a woman it is her natural duty, and not only should she attempt it, but she feels under an obligation to perform well. The differential esteem felt by and for the older carer speaks eloquently of the long and deforming fingers of gender.

Acknowledgements

Acknowledgments to Bradford University Research Committee for a small grant to support this research; to Sarah Hogdson for sharing the interviewing; our colleagues Mike Fisher and Alison Froggart for their methodological and substantive advice, to participants at the Surrey Gender and Ageing symposium for their constructive comments and especially our editors for all their help.

10

GENDER ROLES, EMPLOYMENT AND INFORMAL CARE

*Anne Martin Matthews
and Lori D. Campbell*

The relationship between gender and the provision of care to the frail elderly is typically studied in terms of comparisons between men and women 'caregivers'. In such analyses, women are found to predominate as carers, and to differ from men in terms of the type of care which they provide and the intensity of their involvement. However, these analyses of the intersection of gender and caring frequently convey a rather static view, failing to portray the complex and dynamic relationship between gender and the provision of care to elderly people.

A more process-oriented conceptualization of the relationship between gender and caring can enhance our understanding of how men and women are differentially involved in, and variously affected by, the provision of care to elderly family members. Although such a conceptualization is best achieved using longitudinal or time series data, it can also be realized, albeit to a limited extent, using cross-sectional data which focus on different points or stages in the process. This chapter takes the latter approach. The conceptualization begins with a consideration of what caring is, or, more specifically, what social scientists and researchers understand it to be. The chapter then examines the relationship between gender and caring in terms of taking on the caregiver role; the gendered patterns of involvement in the role; and the consequences or correlates of role involvement. The chapter concludes with a consideration of limitations of the current understanding of the relationship between gender and caring, especially in terms of the relationship between role performance, identity and meaning.

Conceptualizing the caregiver role

Problems of definition pose a considerable obstacle to the understanding of the provision of care to elderly people. As Stone (1991: 724) has noted, 'there is no consensus among researchers, policy makers, service providers, caregivers or care recipients themselves as to what constitutes family caregiving. And the definition of family caregiver varies widely'. Caregivers are variously defined by the types of care provided; by the volume, intensity and duration of assistance; the relationship of the caregiver to the care recipient; and characteristics of the care receiver, such as dementia (Martin Matthews and Rosenthal 1993). Arber and Ginn (1990) distinguish between 'caring' and 'normal' family care by considering qualitative differences in the support and assistance provided by 'carers' and 'helpers'. Rarely is the caring relationship conceptualized in terms of a continuum along which family members move over time, from reciprocal exchanges of help, to the provision of modest levels of assistance and, for some, ultimately to situations requiring intensive levels of care for a highly dependent elderly person (an exception is Taraborrelli 1993). Studies typically consider all types of 'carers' together, or focus on only one point on the continuum, often in terms of the provision of help with activities of daily living (Katz *et al.* 1963).

Due to a lack of longitudinal research, involvement in the caring role frequently appears as chronic or static when, in fact, the provision of care to an older person may be episodic and characterized by 'crisis' events which are resolved permanently, or for a time, only to recur. In addition, researchers frequently define involvement in the caring role in terms of the performance of specific 'tasks'. Such a conceptualization of the caring role neglects important aspects of 'emotion work' (MacRae 1994) often carried out primarily by women and involving the provision of emotional support. These definitional problems substantially complicate the understanding of the relationship between gender and caregiving.

The implications of the concepts researchers and policy makers use in defining caregiving, and how they relate to the understanding of the relationship between caregiving and gender are illustrated by the use of the term 'eldercare'. The term has considerable currency in the private sector because of its assumed parallels with childcare and all that it connotes in terms of issues, programmes and benefits. But the parallels are in fact few. The trajectory of the relationship is far more heterogeneous and unpredictable in the case of eldercare than for childcare. In cases where the development of the child follows a 'normal' and healthy pattern, the provision of childcare is highly regularized in terms of the sequence of responsibilities of the carer, and the anticipated duration of the role. This is not the case for eldercare, where responsibilities may wax and wane in relation to the health or other transitions in the life of the elderly person, and where the anticipated duration of involvement in the carer role is largely unknown. There may also be differences between childcare and eldercare in the number of carers involved (the provision of care to older people may be restricted to one primary carer, or may involve a broader network of kin and friends who function as secondary caregivers). Where several carers are involved there are often complex negotiations and rearrangements to be made.

Childcare and eldercare also vary in their crisis episodes. Illness episodes in children frequently follow a regularized course so that even if the onset of illness cannot be predicted, the 'courses and sequelae' (Avison *et al.* 1993) will typically be experienced as a matter of days rather than weeks or months. Recovery from illness or injury is a lengthy and more complicated process in later life, and employed family members who provide eldercare are far more likely than those providing childcare to require longer periods of time away from paid employment in order to cope with such episodes (Martin Matthews and Rosenthal 1993). Childcare and eldercare also vary in the role of the 'cared for' in setting the definition and expectations of the care. There is, amongst those involved in the provision of care to older people, increasing recognition of the rights of older persons as autonomous decision makers in relation to the care they receive; care arrangements which may be best suited to the needs of the older person may not be compatible with the needs of family members involved in the provision of care. Children typically have no comparable role in determining the care they will receive and accept. Finally, childcare and eldercare differ in terms of the involvement of community-based services in the provision of care. Informal carers not only provide direct assistance to older people; they frequently also 'manage' the care the older person receives through formal service providers (James 1992), in terms of negotiating for and making arrangements on the older person's behalf, monitoring formal service use, and supplementing or bridging between services. The availability and accessibility of community services directly influence the patterns of family involvement in 'eldercare' in a manner not comparable for childcare.

The conceptualization of care of elderly people in terms of eldercare promotes and reinforces an image of older people as inherently dependent. It metaphorically connotes 'care' as equivalent to that given to the child who has not yet achieved the age of majority. In so doing, it fails to acknowledge the important role of reciprocity in patterns of intergenerational relations (Martin Matthews 1993). It promotes and reinforces an image of elderly people only as recipients of care, despite the broad base of gerontological research which documents the prevalence of reciprocal exchanges between elderly people and members of their kin and friendship networks.

Despite these difficulties with the concept of eldercare, the term has become widely used, especially in North America, in discussions of the 'business' of ageing. Various 'national eldercare institutes' have been established in the United States, and the term 'corporate eldercare' is widely used to describe the provision by employers of programmes, benefits and/or services designed to assist employees in caring for elderly family members. It is ironic that the widespread use of a concept which perpetuates images of older people in dependent roles and non-reciprocal relationships should come at a time when the ability of older people to live independently into advanced old age is greater than it has ever been.

Methods and data

To illustrate further the implications of the varying definitions of caregiving for understanding the relationship between gender and caring, this chapter examines several elements of caregiving. In so doing, the chapter reports the results of a Canadian study of employees with responsibilities for care of older family members, defined as aged 65 and over. Over 5,600 men and women involved in paid employment completed postal questionnaires which enquired into their patterns of balancing a range of work and family responsibilities. Although the focus of the study was on employees who provided assistance to an elderly family member at least once in the six months preceding the data collection, employees with childcare responsibilities, and those not involved in providing assistance either to children or to elderly kin provided a comparison group. More detailed information on the methodology of the study is provided in Martin Matthews and Rosenthal (1993) and by Gottlieb *et al.* (1994).

Taking on the role of caregiver

There are significant gender differences in the likelihood of taking on the caregiver role; women predominate among those providing assistance to elderly family members. Data from several national US (Stone *et al.* 1987) and Canadian (Canadian Study of Health and Aging 1994) studies indicate that approximately three-quarters of all informal caregivers are women. However, the picture becomes somewhat more complicated when considering the relationship between gender, employment and informal care. Many carers experience delayed re-entry into the paid labour force because of their caring responsibilities. Others withdraw from the paid labour force for similar reasons. It is estimated that between 9 and 11 per cent of carers relinquish employment because of their caring responsibilities (MacBride-King 1990; Canadian Study of Health and Aging 1994). Women are much more likely than men to withdraw from paid employment for these reasons (Stone *et al.* 1987). Thus studies of employed caregivers potentially overemphasize men's involvement and underrepresent women's involvement in caring for elderly people.

Using various definitional and measurement criteria may yield different estimates of the number of individuals actively engaged in balancing responsibilities for work and for an ageing family member (Martin Matthews and Rosenthal 1993). Such sources of variability become especially important when studying the relationship between gender and taking on the caregiver role. Our data demonstrate that the most inclusive definitions of 'eldercare' magnify men's involvement, while studies more specifically focused on the provision of assistance with the activities of daily living indicate that women provide more care than men. A simple count of all employees who have provided any kind of assistance to an elderly relative in the past six months, regardless of type or frequency of that assistance, indicates little gender difference in the provision of informal care (44 per cent of women employees and 47 per cent of men).

However, if we distinguish between the provision of assistance with the instrumental activities of daily living (such as transport, shopping, laundry, finances and arranging services) and providing personal care (such as assisting with bathing, feeding, toileting, dressing, and administration of medication), gender differences emerge. For this analysis, types of care are categorized as 'instrumental care' and 'personal care' (while recognizing that those providing personal care will usually also assist with instrumental care tasks).

Fourteen per cent of employed women and 8 per cent of employed men in this study are involved in the provision of personal care to an elderly family member. Adopting Stone and Kemper's (1989) criterion of providing assistance with at least two personal care activities, then 8 per cent of the women and 4 per cent of the men are providing personal care. These very stringent definitional measures of what constitutes care corroborate research findings of the greater involvement of women than men in the caring role. The provision of instrumental care presents a rather different profile of the relationship between gender, employment and informal care; 31 per cent of the women and 40 per cent of the men provide only instrumental care to an elderly family member. But research by Matthews and Rosner (1988) suggests that, in comparison to women, men's caregiving styles consist mainly of providing 'back-up', circumscribed and sporadic care.

If a criterion of time spent is used, rather than type of care, in the estimation of who provides informal care, a similar pattern emerges. Arber and Ginn (1990) suggest that the provision of five hours of assistance per week is an important factor in distinguishing between 'carers' and 'helpers'. Just over a quarter of women employees (27 per cent) but a third of the men (33 per cent) provide between one and four hours per week of assistance to older kin. However, when the analysis of prevalence is restricted to those providing five or more hours of assistance per week, the pattern reverses; 13 per cent of the women employees and 8 per cent of the men provide this amount of care.

Not surprisingly, when the prevalence of informal care is estimated either on the basis of type of care (personal versus instrumental) or amount of care (at least five hours of care per week, or less), the broader the operational definition of care, the higher the prevalence estimate (Gorey *et al.* 1992). However, more inclusive definitions increase the estimate of men's involvement in caring more than women's. Hence, how caregiving is conceptualized will directly influence the estimate of gender differences in the provision of informal care.

The relationship between gender and taking on the caregiver role is affected by family structure and class. Our data indicate that men providing personal care are significantly more likely than other men to have no siblings; they are also significantly less likely to have a sibling network of only sisters. Men who provide personal care are almost twice as likely as women who do so to be only children without siblings (11 per cent compared with 6 per cent).

Marital status also influences the relationship between gender, employment and informal care. Although other researchers have found that men who have never married are more likely than married men to be a main carer for a parent (Arber and Ginn 1995a), the Canadian data on employees suggest a different pattern. Amongst male employees, those who have never married are in fact least likely to be providing care, especially personal care, to an elderly family member. Moreover, men are significantly more likely than women who provide personal care to be married and less likely to have never married. Contrary to what had been expected, being single and co-resident with an elderly relative does not increase the likelihood that men will be involved in the provision of care. Indeed, if being single and co-resident with an elderly relative represents a situation of 'caring by default' (Arber and Ginn 1990), then employed women providing personal care are somewhat more likely than employed men to be in these circumstances.

Other structural factors, such as education, income and occupational status may influence whether the role of caregiver is adopted. Examining class differences in co-resident caring, Arber and Ginn (1992) find that working-class men and women provide more care than their middle-class counterparts, and that semi-skilled and unskilled men are more likely to become carers than are other men (and are as likely as women to provide care). The intersection of gender and class suggests that working-class men, especially if they have never left home, may be in a relatively powerless position (compared to their middle-class counterparts) with fewer resources with which to 'resist' the caring role. Middle-class men, with more socioeconomic resources indicative of more power, may be better able to pay for care or have greater influence over others to secure informal assistance. For men, it may be the degree of power they have and their access to resources (particularly financial) which will affect whether they provide care to an elderly parent, or the amount and type of care they provide.

Therefore, care may be provided by default or because men lack the resources or power to resist the caring role; in Finch's terminology (1989: 210) they lack the 'legitimate excuses' to avoid providing care; thus they are unable *not* to care. For women, the expectation that they will provide care to an elderly parent is more normative and therefore more pervasive across socioeconomic groups, although the impact of caring does vary by class (Martin Matthews and Rosenthal 1994).

The intersection between class and gender is important in the interpretation of our data. The likelihood of assuming the role of carer is a function not only of gender, but also of class, especially for men. The relationship is not linear, however, and varies somewhat in terms of measures of occupation and education. Men in managerial and professional positions are underrepresented among employees providing care, especially those providing personal care. Men with the lowest levels of education (less than high school graduation) and those with university postgraduate education are overrepresented among those providing personal care. Thus while some men who provide personal care do represent a well-educated, high income population in managerial or professional occupations, a substantial group of men providing personal care lack the socioeconomic resources which may have enabled them to 'resist' the caring role and associated tasks. They provide personal care because they have no siblings to share or take responsibility for caring; or they may be working-class men with insufficient power and resources to remain outside the caring role, to pay for care, or to influence others to provide care.

Patterns of involvement in the caregiving role

While there is substantial variation by gender in the likelihood of becoming a caregiver, once the role is assumed there are fewer differences between men and women in the patterns of role involvement. There are greater gender differences in relation to the provision of instrumental care and less relating to personal care. Among employed caregivers it is important to remember that over three-quarters of those providing personal care to an elderly family member are women.

There are gender differences in the frequency of tasks performed by carers who only provide instrumental care. Women provide more frequent assistance than men with laundry, transport, shopping, meal preparation and coping with mood swings. Reflecting the findings of previous research on the gendered nature of informal care, men help more frequently than women with home maintenance, managing money and with finances.

Among those providing personal care, there are no gender differences in the frequency of performance of tasks, but some gender variation in the nature of the specific tasks performed. For example, where personal care was provided women were more likely then men to assist with bathing the elderly relative (a task involving half of the men providing personal care but three-quarters of the women). This pattern may reflect Rose and Bruce's observation (Chapter 9) of 'strong feelings about gender boundaries', especially in relation to intimate, personal care. For some kinds of care, it may be unacceptable to the dependent person to have care provided by a man (Arber and Ginn 1995b).

There is some gender difference in the amount of time devoted to the caregiving role. Men average fewer hours of care per week than women, even among those providing the most intensive levels of care. However, the gender difference is not as great as the predominant image of women carers might suggest (Montgomery and McGlinn 1992). Men who provide personal care, and who have principal responsibility for one or more elderly relatives, average 10.9 hours of care per week, compared to 11.8 hours for women in the same circumstance.

Figure 10.1   Job effects of informal care by gender

(a) Personal care – per cent reporting each effect

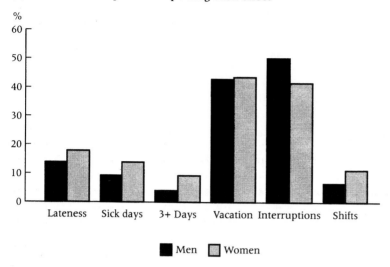

(b) Instrumental care – per cent reporting each effect

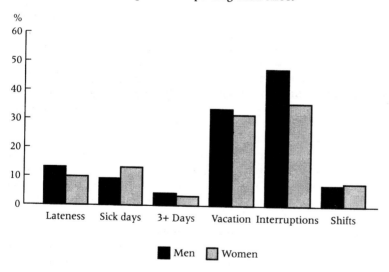

As noted at the beginning of this chapter, the provision of care to elderly family members is often episodic in nature, and characterized by intermittent 'crises'. In addition to the more routine and regularized tasks of care provision,

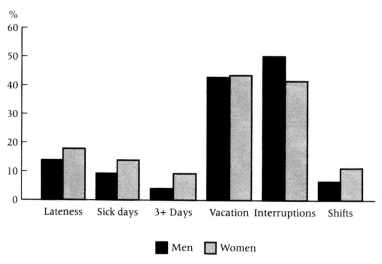

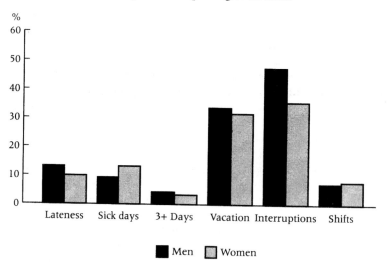

68 per cent of women and men providing personal care report involvement in one or more such episodes in the preceding six months.

Overall these data suggest a highly gendered pattern of involvement in the provision of instrumental assistance to elderly family members. However, for that minority of men who provide personal care, the pattern of role involvement appears to resemble that of women, at least in terms of the nature and frequency of assistance provided.

Consequences of involvement in caregiving roles

For both men and women there are workplace and personal costs associated with involvement in caring roles. These costs include not only effects on the job and longer term career costs, but also personal costs. With respect to job effects, employees were asked whether, in the past six months, family responsibilities had led to: partial absenteeism (arriving late for work or leaving early from work); using sick days when not sick; absences of three or more days because of family responsibilities; using vacation time to attend to family obligations; interrupted work days; or being unable to work their desired shift (Figure 10.1).

Career opportunity costs were measured by asking whether, in the past six months, employees' informal care responsibilities had caused them to: miss business meetings or training sessions; to decline business travel; to miss job-related social events; decline extra projects; decline or not seek a promotion; or to experience difficulty with their manager or supervisor (Figure 10.2). To measure personal costs, employees were asked whether, in the past six months, they had experienced a reduction in time available for the following activities because of informal care responsibilities: volunteer work, leisure activities, continuing education, socializing with friends, housework, or sleeping (Figure 10.3). These 'costs' differ for men and women providing personal care, instrumental care, and for those without such responsibilities (not shown in figures). The assessment of 'cost' differences for men and for women by type of care suggests a complex set of relationships.

The relationship between gender, informal care and consequences for employment differs somewhat for the outcome measures examined here. For some factors, gender differences among those providing personal care to an elderly relative are minimal, for example in the the use of vacation days to deal with family responsibilities and the missing of business trips.

In the majority of cases, however, gender differences are apparent, regardless of the type of informal care provided. Women carers are more likely than men to use sick days to meet their family obligations and are more likely to miss work-related social events. Men are generally more likely than women to report interrupted work days. A major gender difference is seen in relation to promotion (Figure 10.2), with women almost twice as likely to report lost opportunities for promotion because of providing informal care. Unlike many of the more short term job effects examined (Figure 10.1), this kind of response

Figure 10.2   Career opportunity costs of informal care by gender

(a) Personal care – per cent reporting each effect

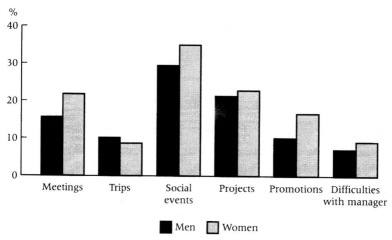

Men   Women

(b) Instrumental care – per cent reporting each effect

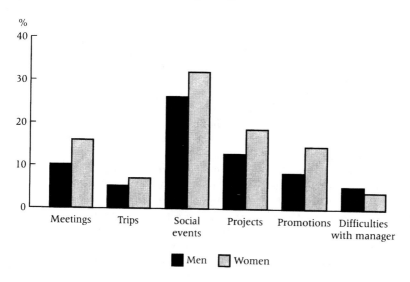

Men   Women

to the need to balance work and family responsibilities has long term consequences for careers and, potentially, for income. Regardless of the type of care they are providing, women are significantly more likely than men to report most of the career opportunity costs indicated in Figure 10.2.

In some cases, gender differences are primarily observed in relation to particular patterns of informal care. In these situations, it is typically women

Figure 10.3   Personal costs of informal care by gender

(a) Personal care – per cent reporting each effect

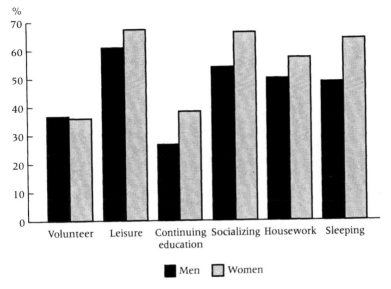

(b) Instrumental care – per cent reporting each effect

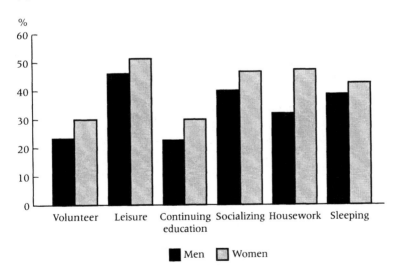

providing personal care who are most likely to report such costs; this is true of absences of three or more days, missing meetings, and not being able to work the desired shift. There are also a very few circumstances in which involvement in more intensive levels of personal care reduces gender differences observable amongst those providing instrumental care. Where this occurs, the effects of providing personal care are comparable for both women and men, whereas the effects are greater for women than men providing instrumental care. This occurs for career opportunity costs (Figure 10.2) such as declining extra work projects, and personal costs (Figure 10.3), involving reductions in voluntarism.

Personal care has a greater impact than instrumental care on employment for both women and men. Women who provide personal care are significantly more likely than women providing instrumental care, or women without informal care responsibilities to report virtually *all* types of job effects, career opportunity costs, and personal costs. Men providing personal care are more likely than those providing instrumental care, or those with no informal care responsibilities, to report a number of workplace and personal costs: the job costs of use of vacation time (Figure 10.1); the career costs related to missed meetings, missed business trips, and declined projects (Figure 10.2); and nearly *all* personal costs (volunteer work, leisure activities, socializing with friends, housework, and sleeping; Figure 10.3).

Overall, both men and women who combine employment and the provision of personal care are significantly more likely to experience job effects, career costs, and personal costs than are their peers who are without informal care responsibilities or those providing only instrumental care. While it is the women providing personal care who experience more (and virtually all) of these job, career, and personal costs, men providing personal care to an elderly relative also experience many of the same costs, although not generally to the same extent as women. 'Mr Wonderful', like his unheralded female counterpart, pays a price at the office and on the factory floor.

The application of knowledge of gender differences

The issues addressed in this chapter, and the empirical data used to illustrate them, corroborate the findings of other researchers as to the importance of gender when the caregiver role is taken on, and add to our understanding of the complex relationship between gender and caregiving in terms of actual patterns of role involvement, and how issues of gender may become more blurred and diffuse once the caregiver role moves along the continuum to involve very intensive and heavy levels of personal care. However, the analysis of gender issues among this group of caregivers also reflects a realization about the worrisome potential for misinterpretation of data which focus virtually exclusively on women's caring roles. It is a potential which is characteristic of much applied research in the social sciences, and warrants further explanation here.

Because this research was undertaken with the cooperation of nine Canadian companies, the first stage of data dissemination involved providing feedback reports to each employer. Each report profiled company-specific as well as general issues involving employees and their balance of responsibilities, relating to their employment, to children and/or to elderly family members, or for home life in general. In each of the reports, and as emphasized in this chapter, it was abundantly clear that women were significantly more likely than men to report responsibilities for care of elderly family members; women spent more time in the provision of this care, and were far more likely than men to be involved in the provision of types of care known to reflect greater frailty and dependence of the care recipient.

The feedback reports emphasized that employees with responsibilities for care of at least one elderly family member were significantly more likely than employees without such responsibilities to report all types of job effects and career opportunity costs. Furthermore, they clearly indicated that women were significantly more likely than men to report these costs, largely because of their predominance as carers, especially in the provision of the most demanding kinds of personal care. Individuals who combined responsibilities for children and for elderly family members were especially likely to report such costs, and women again predominated amongst this group of employees (Martin Matthews and Rosenthal 1993).

Social science research has an important role to play in advancing societal recognition of the carework by women (Kyle 1993; Nelson 1994), and the obstacles they face to career advancement because of their multiple role responsibilities. This task of communication was actively played by members of this research team. At another level, however, members of the research team felt considerable anxiety concerning the potential for misapplication of research findings. Clearly the data provided yet further empirical evidence of the costs which women bear in the workplace, and of the fact that employer policies and managerial attitudes are not uniformly supportive of the delicate balance between work and family life. By establishing that reality within the context of each occupational setting, members of the research team saw themselves as advocating more progressive policies or positive management attitudes. Nevertheless, a subtext of these findings might also read as 'caregiving is a women's issue' and 'women with informal care responsibilities are a company liability'. Our research findings highlighted the costs of the interrupted workdays, the use of sick days for family reasons, the absenteeism resulting from tardy arrivals and early departures from work, the inability to take on extra projects, the difficulties with managers, and the declining of career advancement – and emphasized these especially in relation to women.

Such findings allow the calculation of the potential 'costs' of women employees to their employers, and could be misused, if they become a rationale for discouraging the hiring, training and promotion of women because of potential disruptions associated with their caring responsibilities. Our data demonstrated that women experience these job and personal costs at all levels of the occupational hierarchy; indeed, amongst those providing care to elderly family members, women in management and professional occupations were and service occupations to report job effects, career opportunity costs and personal costs (Martin Matthews and Rosenthal 1994).

An aim of our study was to consider whether women report more of these kinds of costs simply because they are more likely to provide care to elderly family members. The data presented in this chapter suggest that the 'costs of caring' are not equitably borne by men and women. Costs are greater among, but not exclusive to, women carers. As men become involved in caring roles they too experience many of these costs, although to a lesser extent than women. It is important to recognize men's involvement (and its associated costs) so that it is not only women who are seen as the 'less reliable' or 'more problematic' employees.

Conclusions and caveats

Gender differences emerge across all aspects of the conceptualization of caregiving as process, but are especially noteworthy in terms of taking on the role and in the consequences or correlates of involvement in caregiving. The broader the operational definition of care adopted, the higher the estimate of prevalence of informal care by men. Many factors intersect with gender to determine the likelihood of taking on the role of carer; these include marital status, nature of sibling network and class (as reflected by income, education and occupational status).

The most striking feature of the relationship between gender and patterns of caregiving is the overwhelming predominance of women as providers of personal care. The relationship between gender, informal care and employment costs is complex. It varies somewhat according to the type of care provided and the particular outcomes, in terms of job, career and personal costs. The long term consequences associated with not seeking promotion or career advancement are, however, particularly pronounced for women involved in the provision of personal care. To paraphrase McMullin's observation in Chapter 3, this analysis of gender, employment and informal care suggests that personal relations, marital relations and class relations are the gendered processes through which involvement in caring for older people occurs.

Despite the plethora of recent research on the caregiving role, several essential issues remain unanswered in the consideration of the relationship between gender, employment and informal care. Rose and Bruce (Chapter 9) discuss the intersection of ageing, ethnicity and gender with reference to the caring role. The role of ethnicity is rarely acknowledged in the examination of gender, employment and informal care. In this study, foreign-born men were significantly more likely than foreign-born women to have an elderly relative but not be providing either instrumental or personal care. Cultural norms involving the provision of care to elderly relatives are little known and not well understood. This is a significant oversight in countries such as Canada which have in recent years been characterized by high rates of immigration based on policies of family reunification. Indeed, in this study, 24 per cent of the men and 21 per cent of the women surveyed were born outside Canada.

In addition, little is known about the relationship between the provision of assistance and the performance of specific tasks, and the meaning of these in relation to a perceived identity as a caregiver or eldercare provider. This relationship (between performance and identity and meaning) is especially critical in examining the relationship between gender and involvement in the caring role, for example in helping to explain the finding that men report high levels of involvement in the provision of intimate, personal care to parents and parents-in-law (especially mothers), despite cultural taboos concerning such activities. We do not know what men mean when they say they are 'involved' in this type of care. Does it mean that they 'helped' their spouse or partner undertaking this role, but that she had primary responsibility for performance of the task? Does it reflect a reality wherein men identify with the responsibility but not with the actual execution of the tasks associated with the responsibility? Such a point of view was expressed by one man who identified himself as a caregiver: 'My wife does most of it. It is a joint effort' (Vonhof 1991: 18).

Do men carers assume a proactive, responsible role in relation to the tasks which comprise caregiving, especially personal care? Or is their involvement sporadic and episodic, coming only when, through a process of default, there is no one else available? This chapter has emphasized the complex and multidimensional character of the relationship between gender and the provision of care to elderly relatives. The meaning of this relationship in terms of the lived experience of these men and women carers and care recipients remains, as yet, to be ascertained.

Acknowledgments

The data reported in this chapter were collected as part of a study of 'Work and Family', conducted by the Work and Eldercare Research Group of CARNET (The Canadian Aging Research Network). Funding of this project was from the Canadian Ministry of Science and Technology through its Networks of Centres of Excellence Program.

11

GENDER AND ELDER ABUSE

Terri Whittaker

Abuse of older people is not a new problem but one which has existed in various forms and settings for a long time (Thomas 1978; Stearns 1986). Contemporary interest in the problem of elder abuse has arisen in the context of earlier recognition of wife battering and child abuse and shares several important features. First, the process of recognition of elder abuse as a discrete social problem has been slow in Britain, though there is clearly greater public and professional awareness within the USA and Canada where considerable resources have been devoted to the topic both in research and policy terms (Ogg 1993). Second, there has been much debate and controversy concerning definitions and conceptualizations of elder abuse, with a consequent lack of consistency in terms of research findings on incidence and prevalence. Third and most significantly, strenuous efforts have been made to portray elder abuse as a product of either carer stress/pathology and/or dysfunctional families, with a consequent underplaying of the role of men as abusers and an obscuring of issues of gender and power within the family and wider society.

This chapter questions the way that elder abuse has been represented as a problem of carer stress and/or family violence and points to the definitional, methodological and theoretical weaknesses in the literature. The marked absence of studies which treat age, gender and power as fundamental social divisions rather than as variables within established malestream categories of analysis is noted. An attempt is made to illustrate how feminist theory and methodology could be developed to provide a fully gendered account of elder abuse which recognizes the interconnections between age, gender, power and other forms of social division and oppression.

The final section of the chapter looks at existing policy and considers how a feminist analysis of elder abuse might be formulated to situate the problem of elder abuse within the wider social structure, recognizing the wide range of situations and settings in which abuse occurs and questioning the wisdom of grouping so many types and forms of abuse within the broad category of elder abuse. Existing policy directives aimed at reducing carer stress and the underlying assumption that this will reduce actual or potential abuse are considered critically.

Elder abuse: Methodological and theoretical problems

The last decade has witnessed a flurry of research and academic publications on elder abuse, mainly from the USA (Sengstock and Liang 1982; Eastman 1984; Phillips 1986; Pillemer and Wolf 1986; Quinn and Tomita 1986; Godkin *et al.* 1989; Pritchard 1992; Bennett and Kingston 1993; Decalmer and Glendenning 1993). This has occurred in the context of rapid growth in the elderly population and concern about the changing nature of the family (Phillipson 1993a).

Early research relating to elder abuse focused on the characteristics and circumstances of 'victims' who were typically physically and/or mentally frail older women. More recently the discourse on elder abuse has shifted towards an orthodoxy in which the gendered nature of the phenomenon is increasingly obscured within obsessive searches for consensus over definition and prevalence. In this context, various individual or family based models of 'inadequate caregiving' and/or of 'family pathology' have dominated at the explanatory level.

The notion of gender relations implies an interconnectedness with other social divisions and phenomena. Hanmer and Hearn (1994) argue that violence and abuse are directly connected with gender relations. From this perspective, a fully gendered account of elder abuse would need to treat gender and elder abuse through its interrelations with other social divisions, other oppressions and other identities. Of particular importance here would be exploration of the relationship between gender and age (Arber and Ginn 1991a). Feminist analysis is well placed to develop such an account, because gender is basic to the understanding of violence and abuse. Though feminist analysis could make a valuable contribution in developing existing theory and methodology, there is a curious lack of such analysis within the literature. How far this is a reflection of the fact that feminist theorists have tended to neglect age relations is an important question.

Definitional disarray: Contested terrain and competing realities

Social theory and associated definitions are not constructed in a social or political vacuum. Parton (1985) notes the processes by which definitions of child abuse serve the interests of particular professions and give new momentum to 'orthodox' research and policy formulations. The success of the women's movement in acquiring and challenging such 'orthodox' knowledge and in transforming it through feminist theory and methodology is well documented (Kelly 1988).

A review of available US and UK research reveals that the process of reaching definitional agreement about elder abuse is fraught with difficulties and that certain groups of professionals and academics have been heavily influential. The 1980s saw many definitions of elder abuse and a widespread recognition that they lacked clarity and precision (Hudson 1986; Pillemer and Finkelhor 1988; Wolf 1988; Filinson and Ingman 1989; Stevenson 1989; Wolf and Pillemer 1989). The main problems identified focused on which criteria to include or exclude in various definitions of abuse and on whether elder abuse is different from other forms of family violence.

These difficulties have been attributed to differences in emphasis and perspective among investigators, with some proposing typologies of elder abuse and others conceptualizing on the basis of reasons for abuse. How far these difficulties are also a product of the assumption that theory derives from definition rather than the reverse is a question which needs to be answered.

Incidence and prevalence: Another false trail?

The obsession with definitions of elder abuse is mirrored in the concern with incidence and prevalence. Prevalence studies are highly political activities, particularly in the light of 'new knowledge' that women are also abusers. As yet there is no consensus about how common elder abuse is. There has been no major study of the prevalence or incidence of elder abuse in Britain, while American studies have been heavily criticized for the methodological problems of the available research. The unreliability of statistics which vary from state to state, from definition to definition and from data source to data source has been widely noted (Decalmer and Glendenning 1993). The prevalence of elder abuse in the USA was first estimated at 4 per cent of the elderly population (Block and Sinnott 1979) but the research methodology underpinning this study has since been widely discredited. There is now a general acceptance that prevalence rates are lower than this (Ogg 1993) and that the substantial discrepancies among estimates of incidence and prevalence make it impossible to compare results meaningfully (Weiss 1988).

Prevalence studies are underpinned by theories, definitions, conceptualiz- ations and categories of elder abuse which are themselves gendered. Policies and procedures of agencies, such as social services departments, are also gendered and present gendered understandings of abuse which inform and direct policies and practices; these in turn inform theories, definitions and conceptualizations of abuse. Collecting statistics on elder abuse is therefore not the objective, value-free process that it is commonly held to be (Milner 1993).

Milner (1993) stresses that in child abuse, as in other forms of abuse, men and women are treated differently; the role of men as perpetrators is obscured in the investigative process due to the way differing categories of abuse are combined. In this context, the claim that women and men abuse older people in almost equal numbers (Pillemer and Finkelhor 1988) needs to be treated with caution and the methodologies underpinning such studies subjected to rigorous examination. The few studies which have separated differing types of abuse have discovered statistically significant gender differences; men are more likely to physically and/or sexually abuse older women, while women are more likely to report feeling stress and neglecting the older person (Homer and Gilleard 1990; Holt 1993). Although it is by no means clear that violence, abuse and neglect are aspects of a single phenomenon, these findings can be interpreted in ways which neutralize the debate around elder abuse and discourage a gendered analysis.

Questions about why men and women are likely to engage in differing forms of elder abuse or neglect require gendered answers which cannot be obtained by adding gender to malestream social theories of child or spouse abuse. It is likely that, given differences in the way men and women perceive and talk about violence and abuse, in the amount of time men and women spend caring and in the types of tasks undertaken, women may be more exposed to caregiving stress and more ready to talk about it. The gendered nature of caring and the differing expectations and attitudes held by men and women towards caring for older people may lead women carers to report abusive incidents more readily. This may result in neglect or inadequate caregiving being more prominent than other forms of abuse in informing the construction of theory, methodology, policy and practice.

There is a danger that elder abuse will continue to be conceptualized mainly as a problem of stress, inadequate caregiving or, where these approaches cannot be used to explain extreme acts of violence to older women, then psychopathology of the abuser becomes the causal explanation. MacPherson (1990) argues that much elder abuse remains hidden and suggests that this is probably the more violent end of the abuse spectrum. As yet, we do not know how much elder abuse there is or what types are most common but it is clear that framing the problem in terms of stress and/or inadequate care invites certain types of responses and discourages others.

Elder abuse and social theory

The definitional and methodological disarray which underpins the elder abuse literature is arguably a product of inadequate and/or inappropriate theoretical development and an assumption that definition comes before theory. To date there has been no specific attempt to develop a theory specific to elder abuse but rather a tendency to fit age and the phenomenon of elder abuse into various malestream theories of carer stress/inadequacy or family pathology, the assumption being that the life experiences of older people in general and older women in particular can be explained using the same theoretical frameworks as for younger men and women. The three main theoretical approaches – situational stress, individual pathology of the abuser and family violence – are briefly outlined.

Situational stress

Until recently, most research attention has focused on the characteristics of the victims of elder abuse, creating a stereotypical picture of the nature of old age. The classic victim of elder abuse has been painted by various British, Canadian and American researchers as:

1   female aged over 75;
2   living at home with adult carer/s;
3   physically and/or mentally impaired;
4   roleless; previous roles as wife/mother/caregiver lost;
5   isolated and fearful

(Tomlin 1989; Bennett 1990)

This profile of the victim of abuse is associated with liberal explanations of elder abuse which assume a direct correlation between biological ageing and dependency (Phillips 1986: 198). The situational or 'carer stress' model is derived from research on child abuse, in which abuse is explained in terms of the dependency of the victim and how this causes stress for the carer, whose gender is left unidentified. Though studies underpinned by this perspective generally agree that the overwhelming majority of victims are older women (quoted in McCreadie 1991: 21), gender has generally been included as a variable and not used as a central category of analysis.

It is thus not surprising that, despite contradictory research findings, the situational stress model, which is underpinned by stereotypical notions of later life as dependency as well as a concern with preserving the family, has had huge appeal for professionals. The latter, whilst not condoning abuse, have tended to downplay its gendered character and to focus on interventionist strategies aimed at reducing carer stress. Though no attempt is made to define the concept of carer stress, there is a commonsense appeal about the model which implies that everyone knows what it is. Where the notion of stress cannot be used to explain all acts of abuse, then psychopathology usually becomes the causal explanation; here attention shifts to the personality traits of the abuser, whose gender is not considered relevant.

Pathology of abusers

In the mid-1980s, the focus of attention on elder abuse shifted away from 'granny battering', with its specific gender connotations, towards gender neutral notions of 'inadequate care giving'. This shift served to inhibit understanding of the gendered nature of elder abuse and to perpetuate malestream sociological ideas about the ungendered individual within the family (Hanmer 1990). New research drawing on theories of family pathology challenged the idea of a close association between abuse and the physical and/or the mental state of the victim, suggesting that the characteristics and circumstances of the perpetrators may be more important risk indicators (Pillemer and Wolf 1986; Homer and Gilleard 1990).

The concept of 'inadequate care' which is underpinned by a model of a stressed and/or pathological abuser was introduced and facilitated this shift. Attempts were made to identify the predisposing factors leading to elder abuse, with researchers emphasizing the inadequate personality types of ungendered carers and/or their dependency on their care recipient, or on alcohol or other drugs. From this perspective, there is nothing inherently violent about the family, which is assumed to conform to an ideal model of harmony and complementarity; violence or abuse occur when carers are personally inadequate. The notion of lack of intention to abuse is used to bolster and legitimate compassionate or supportive forms of intervention as opposed to those which control or coerce. Denial of intention is also used to preserve the autonomy of the family, which serves to obscure further the gendered nature of the phenomenon and to excuse and justify abusive behaviours (Fulmer and O'Malley 1987).

Once again there is no attempt to explicate underlying theories or their value base. Issues of power and politics are notable by their absence and the question of the appropriateness of various models of individual/family pathology as a tool for understanding elder abuse is not raised. Earlier ways of seeing and thinking about elder abuse as a form of 'granny battering' have been dismissed in favour of a new orthodoxy; this holds that elder abuse is much more complex, relating to the nature of the interpersonal relationship between victims and carers.

Elder abuse and family violence

The interest among researchers in the nature and extent of the relationship between elder abuse and other forms of family violence is growing apace. Elder abuse is said to occur in a context of family relations and therefore, it is argued, more attention needs to be paid to the literature relating to child and spouse abuse (Pillemer and Suitor 1988). Some writers have argued that elder abuse should be seen as a part of the spectrum of domestic abuse which affects all ages (Department of Health SSI 1992), whilst others have sought to establish a special category for elder abuse and associated programmes of assessment and intervention (Finkelhor and Pillemer 1988).

The growing interest in domestic violence in general, and child abuse and spouse abuse in particular, is likely to become increasingly dominant in the discourse on elder abuse. However, as with early research and debates on child abuse, the interest is confined to certain liberal and conservative theories of family violence which are often not made explicit, whilst their utility for explaining or understanding elder abuse remains unquestioned. The growing interest in the family is not about making the gender and age significance of abuser and abused more explicit or about exposing the problems of sexual politics inherent in elder abuse. Instead, the research reflects a growing anxiety about the nature of the family and a concern to enshrine and safeguard 'normal' family relationships.

Five major explanations rooted in theories of family violence are examined in the research. They are:

1 pathology of abuser – intra-individual dynamics;
2 cycle of violence – violence transmitted between generations;
3 dependency – of abused and/or abuser;
4 isolation – limited social networks/denial of access;
5 external stress – unemployment, bereavement, inadequate community care, low income, poor housing.

(Pillemer 1986)

Pillemer and Suitor (1988: 127), reviewing the literature associated with these themes, argue: 'These factors may directly precipitate domestic violence against the elderly. That is *families* that have one of these characteristics may be at greater risk of elder abuse' (my emphasis).

What is crucial here is the focus on the family rather than on particular individuals who may have abused or been abused. Indeed the literature is now beginning to be peppered with references to *'abusive families'* (Godkin *et al.* 1989) as systems or sets of interrelationships which are not functioning properly. Thus elder abuse becomes a *symptom* of what is wrong with certain families and the personality traits and behaviour of both victims and abusers are studied, however widely they vary.

Another twist to the tale of the 'problem relative' or family (Pillemer and Finkelhor 1989) lies in the notion of the 'cycle of violence'. Some commentators argue that elder abuse is directly related to the fact that perpetrators were themselves products of domestic violence which has become learned behaviour and normative for them (Fulmer and O'Malley 1987). The child abuse literature has shown how dangerous these ideas are and pointed to the way they feed myths about 'pathological' families and fuel class and race stereotypes to the point where abusers have been known to tell their victims that abuse is quite normal (Nelson 1987: 48).

The idea that perpetrators abuse because they were themselves abused says nothing about those who were abused in childhood who do not subsequently abuse others. Not only does the cycle of violence notion have a spurious liberal appeal by obscuring the gendered nature of elder abuse; it also absolves the abuser of responsibility, prompting compassionate and therapeutic responses and legitimating the role of professionals. At the same time, it implies that abuse only occurs in dysfunctional families and affirms that there is nothing wrong with the wider society.

Towards a gendered analysis of elder abuse

An adequate theoretical base

It is necessary to develop an adequate theoretical base for understanding elder abuse. Explanatory theory is especially important in the area of social problems because if we can provide an account of how the phenomenon identified as needing action is caused, it is in principle possible to do something about it. The preceding review of research literature reveals a range of normative accounts of elder abuse as a symptom of individual or family malfunctioning which, it is implied, is remediable through medical and/or rehabilitative and supportive strategies of intervention.

This health/welfare model of elder abuse dominates policy and practice formulations and has been widely accepted by many professionals working in the field. However, we cannot assume that conceptualizations of social problems which are readily accepted and legitimated are necessarily any more objective and scientific than alternative explanations (Parton 1985). Similar types of health/welfare models of child abuse which dominated debates 20 years ago have been widely criticized and successfully challenged by other explanatory models. These locate the problem within the wider social structure and provide fully gendered accounts as the basis for understanding and action (Kelly 1988).

Hanmer and Hearn (1994) note that fully gendered research on abuse is the exception rather than the rule in the USA. It is perhaps not surprising then that ungendered and individualistic or family based models of analysis, which fit the lives of older people in general and older women in particular into existing categories of analysis, dominate the elder abuse literature. Though feminist theorists have incorporated gender relations as fundamental categories of analysis, they have been slow to consider relationships between age and gender in relation to abuse.

An adequate feminist theory of elder abuse must move beyond health/welfare conceptualizations of the problem to develop a theory in which age and gender and the relationships between them and other social divisions are given equal importance. The lives and experiences of older women should not be subsumed within constructs or categories of analysis which are assumed to be equally applicable to younger and older men and women. It is beyond the scope of this chapter to develop such theory but a brief outline of some important aspects of such an undertaking will be given.

The treatment of power

In the UK, feminist work on violence and abuse towards women and children did not start with notions of stress, inadequate carers, or pathological individuals or families. Instead such work began from a theoretical perspective which focused on oppression, exploitation and the dominance of men over women, both in the family and in society in general. From this perspective, men's power and domination was seen as a central problem and the potential for violence and abuse was seen as fundamental to gender and power in all social relationships.

To date, this type of analysis has not been applied in research on elder abuse or used as a tool to enhance our understanding of the nature of the social relationships between men and older women. Indeed, the discovery that women abuse too and do have power over their victims has been interpreted in ways which preclude such analysis (Pillemer and Wolf 1986; Pillemer and Suitor 1988). A feminist analysis of elder abuse, whilst recognizing the gendered nature of inequality, would have to acknowledge women's capacity for violence and recognize that the issue of power is more problematic and less fixed than previously imagined. The connections between relations of age, gender and power would be central categories of analysis and the notion of power would require a different treatment.

This means treating power like age and gender relations, as something fluid, rather than fixed and monolithic, as something which varies according to what it is in relation to or with. For example the nature and extent of power held by a white woman at any point in time may vary according to her position in relation to her husband, her child, older women, younger women, black women, health, economic status and so forth. In respect of elder abuse, this leads to a concern with how power operates in different contexts. It could also lead to an exploration of abuse in terms of power among different women as well as of the limits of power between women and men.

From this perspective, literature which points to the provoking and controlling behaviours of non-compliant dependent victims, illustrated in statements such as 'the care giver is seen as being driven to a sense of helplessness, rage and frustration' (Decalmer and Glendenning 1993: 15), need careful scrutiny. There is an alternative to seeing such behaviours as indicators of carer stress; it may be more useful to see them as attempts by older men and women to struggle against and resist the larger sociopolitical context of age, gender and power inequality within their personal relationships, which may be with both men and women. Instead of problematizing the biology of later life, a recognition of the socially constructed aspects of dependency which young and older women experience, albeit differently, could be used to develop a better understanding of elder abuse and to challenge dominant stereotypes of older people as a burden and passive recipients of care.

Methodology and empowerment

Feminist critiques of social science methodology have generally focused on sexist bias in research literature from the perspective of white, middle-class, heterosexual, academic feminists (Stanley and Wise 1990). Though some attempts have been made to redress this bias by taking the perspective of black and lesbian women, there is a noticeable absence of a critical perspective from the standpoint of older women (Macdonald and Rich 1984). Consequently, there is an urgent need for a feminist critique of social science methods in relation to the experiences of various groupings of older women.

As yet the voices of survivors of elder abuse have not been heard above those of informal carers or paid experts, so we know very little about the social context in which abused older people live or about their wishes or needs and the strategies they employ to redress power imbalances and fight back. Participative research methods which enable older women to survive abuse and facilitate 'talk and tell' responses are to be encouraged, but must be used responsibly and reflexively to minimize potential exploitation and/or harm (Kelly et al. 1994). Such approaches must be underpinned by theories which recognize the structural inequalities associated with being older and a woman in our society. In particular, older women are likely to have more social and economic difficulties than men in leaving abusive situations (Taylor and Ford 1983; Glendinning 1987; Walker 1987). Thus frail and dependent older women may be more reluctant to disclose abuse or participate in the research process than their male counterparts.

Opie (1992) argues that there are three ways in which women are empowered through participation in research processes: through gaining knowledge and information needed to act; through helping to make a social issue visible; and through the therapeutic effect of re-evaluating their experience. Though all of these forms of empowerment are in theory applicable to women survivors of elder abuse and there is an urgent need for such principles to be extended to research on the experiences of older women, there are a number of potential problems which need to be considered.

First, substantial numbers of survivors of elder abuse may be physically and/or mentally frail and thus less able to evaluate and act on their experiences. In this context, supportive methods of validation and advocacy may be important dimensions of feminist research on elder abuse (Dobash and Dobash 1992). Listening to and validating the feelings and experiences of older women and insisting on their rights to adequate information and independent advocacy, where relevant, may help them overcome difficulties associated with disclosure, including fear of stigma and of institutionalization. Phillipson (1993b) points to the crucial role of advocacy in highlighting injustices which would otherwise remain hidden and to the importance of such an approach as a way of responding to intergenerational conflict.

Feil (1993) has developed a technique for communicating with vulnerable older people and validating their experiences. Such an approach may prove useful from a methodological perspective; it may facilitate disclosure and help researchers to enable older women to express their thoughts and feelings in a form which renders their story credible to those who have responsibility for processing allegations of abuse. As things stand, much of the data from victims in existing research findings has been discounted as unreliable on the grounds of mental impairment (Pillemer and Finkelhor 1988; Homer and Gilleard 1990). An empowering methodology would assert that it is possible to listen to and validate the voices of frail older women and would search for ways and means to ensure that older women's rights were protected.

A methodological approach to elder abuse which attempts to connect age and gender relations would be concerned with the balance of power among older women as members of a marginalized group, and with how this connects to their relationship with other groups and the wider patriarchal society. This means developing methods which recognize the differing experiences among women as well as the connection between men and women and other social divisions, other oppressions and other identities. In this context, it is important to be aware of simplistic notions of participation and empowerment which mask aspects of the power and responsibility of the researcher.

A feminist methodology of elder abuse is thus both a practical and an academic endeavour in that it requires a theoretical, epistemological and methodological framework which hears and validates older women's experiences as the 'other' and relates this to the wider social structure. The current fixation in elder abuse research with large scale prevalence studies, with telephone and postal questionnaires and with comparing prevalence rates is antithetical to the building of knowledge of this kind. There is thus an urgent need to challenge such approaches and develop alternative methodologies, but the presumed benefits of qualitative methods to participants have to be questioned and the potential for harm taken seriously and addressed. Sharing knowledge and information whilst raising awareness may not be experienced as empowering to those older women who find that disclosure results in their being removed to residential care. Fonow and Cook (1991: 8) note that 'a well crafted quantitative study may be more useful to policy makers and cause less harm to women than a poorly crafted qualitative one'.

Elder abuse and social policy

The ideological, theoretical and methodological debates surrounding elder abuse have mirrored those about child abuse, with certain forms of liberal malestream theory dominating debate and policy formulation (Parton 1985). In this context, it is not surprising that agencies charged with responsibility for elder abuse cases have adopted policies and procedures based on normative versions of the family. Models of individual or family pathology may have very little relevance to elder abuse and are certainly not transferable wholesale (Decalmer and Glendenning 1993).

To date, policy initiatives on elder abuse have taken their lead from research and methodologies which are underpinned by dominant ideologies about the family and conceptualizations of abuse as resulting from biological dependency or carer stress. Hence policy developments in Britain have mainly been focused on the needs of carers as a means of reducing carer stress. The underlying assumption, that reducing stress will reduce abuse and thus keep the family intact, has not been tested rigorously. Studies have shown that the link between stress and abuse is a somewhat tenuous one (Homer and Gilleard 1990); other studies have indicated that, despite increases in respite and day care services for carers and the expressed wish of many abused older women to remain in their own homes, abuse continues and a sizeable number do enter residential care (Department of Health SSI 1992).

This is not to argue against support services for carers, especially where it is clear that they will be effective in reducing stress and/or abuse. However, it is important to question the notion of causation implicit in the underlying conceptualization of elder abuse as predominantly a problem of carer or family stress/inadequacy. Given the wide variety of situations and forms of elder abuse, it may be that there are many different social problems beneath the umbrella category of elder abuse. We simply do not know if providing support services for carers or families is the best way of reducing abuse or if all types and forms of abuse are equally responsive to similar policy interventions.

Given these uncertainties it is important to question the way in which the problem of elder abuse has been defined and the underlying assumptions of the models which underpin policy and practise interventions. The way a social problem is defined will shape the nature of social policies devised to address it. The defining of elder abuse as a problem of carer or family stress/pathology has had enormous appeal for professionals from a range of disciplines involved in the regulation of family life. Thus the increasing professionalization and medicalization of elder abuse needs to be treated with caution and the vested interests of professions examined critically.

The literature from the child abuse field charts the huge growth in academic, professional and therapeutic interventions and also demonstrates that they have done little to reduce risk (Parton 1985). Of related importance is the need to guard against the continuation of service-led responses to older people who have been or may be abused. Service-led, as opposed to needs-led, assessment and provision has tended to dominate both health and social care agency responses to older people; as a result, their needs are framed in terms of mainly practical, rehabilitative or support services, while their social, emotional and psychological problems, as well as issues of power and dependency in the caring relationship, are ignored.

Reducing the problem of elder abuse to individual and/or family defects excludes the possibility of a social theory of elder abuse which takes account of the long history of abuse in settings other than the family (Phillipson 1993a). There is an implicit assumption that the wider social structure is unproblematic and that the problem can and should be solved by experts in the field rather than by other means. Of particular relevance here is the law in relation to elder abuse, and the lack of any real debate about the criminal aspects of such abuse. A feminist analysis of elder abuse will need to guard against the dangers inherent in the medicalization of later life and the decriminalization of elder abuse. To rule out coercive policy interventions or legal processes is to give a very clear message to society that abuse of older people in general and older women in particular is not a cause for concern.

A feminist analysis of elder abuse should start with the recognition that abuse cannot be divorced from the social context in which it occurs, and should question the selective claiming and framing of the problem of elder abuse as a product of carer stress and/or family pathology. An alternative construction needs to locate the phenomenon within the patriarchal (as opposed to the pathological) family and its relationship to the state and various social systems therein. This type of analysis will make explicit the tensions within the family and expose the fluid and changing nature of power between men and women in the family, and between the family and the state over who should provide care for older people.

Such an approach will make the connections between gender, age, power and poverty, and will seek to articulate the nature of the tensions and oppressions inherent in the relationship between carer and cared for, whilst at the same time recognizing power differentials and any potential for abuse which may exist. By making explicit the tensions within the family, and between the family and state, and by balancing the voice of the carer with that of the cared for, it becomes possible to question dominant forms of social problem construction; stereotypes which portray older people as burdens and carers as saints may then be challenged and policy changes advocated which place more practical and material resources at the disposal of both carers and cared for.

From this perspective, elder abuse is more complex than carer stress or family pathology. Thus policies focused on supporting carers are unlikely to solve the problem but may function to obscure important issues of age, gender, power, dependence and poverty within the wider social structure. Economic independence for older people in general and older women in particular is crucial to the prevention of abuse in later life. Ageing societies are primarily female societies and ageism and sexism combine to produce a socially constructed dependence in later life in which the feminization of poverty is a key feature (Walker 1987). Any adequate analysis of elder abuse must take account of the social structural position of older women in our society and how this relates to their position within the family and the resources they have at their disposal to resist abusive behaviours.

Adequate legislation which states unequivocally that abuse of older people is unacceptable is also crucial to effective policy and practice interventions, as are adequately resourced community care policies which set minimum standards of care and provide for both carers and cared for. Current community care policy which forces more and more older people into reliance on already overstretched and underresourced systems of family or informal care, which are themselves gendered, can only increase the risk of abuse, especially for the very old and frail, who are predominantly women (Department of Health SSI 1992). More state support and less dependence on the family is also preferred by older people (Finch 1989; McGlone and Cronin 1994).

Conclusion

This chapter has questioned the dominant explanatory models of elder abuse and pointed to the extensive problems inherent in existing research, policy and practice. There is a need to shift the focus away from explanatory models based on individual stress/inadequacy or family violence, with the associated concern with definitions, incidence and prevalence, towards the development of a social model of elder abuse. As with child abuse and wife battering, feminist theory and methodology have a valuable role to play in the development of alternative definitions and analysis of this important phenomenon, making issues of age, gender, power and poverty and the connections between them central to the analysis. From alternative definitions, methodologies and explanations come alternative forms of policy, planning and intervention. The way a problem is defined shapes the nature of the solution. Those involved in the field of elder abuse and feminist research need to engage with the necessary process of problem construction, deconstruction and reconstruction.

12

GENDER AND SOCIAL SUPPORT NETWORKS IN LATER LIFE

Anne Scott and G. Clare Wenger

Informal networks are the framework for social interaction. Social networks consist of all those people with whom we have ongoing relationships and it is through such networks that individual people are linked into groups and society. Because the idea of a network emphasizes relationships among people rather than groups or institutions, it is a particularly suitable tool in the search for understanding the social ageing process (where relationships are central) and how this relates to gender.

Everyone has a social network and within virtually every network there is a *support network*. This consists of all those available, or perceived by the person to be available, to provide emotional support, companionship, instrumental help and advice on a day to day basis. Some kinds of support are part of everyday life – the sharing of domestic tasks in a household, routine borrowing and monitoring of risks among neighbours, talking with friends about joys and sorrows. Other kinds are called on only in particular circumstances such as illness or emergencies. Different members of the network may provide different kinds of support, depending on their relationship to the person and constraints of time, distance and abilities.

The functioning of one's support network is related to the quality of life. A review of the literature (Wenger 1992a) found that friendship, confidant relationships, social support, marital status and social isolation, as well as variables involving health, personal resources and type of neighbourhood were all related to morale in old age.

Most of the population aged 65 and over are active and healthy. However, with advancing age, illness and disability become more common. Arthritis and heart disease head the list of longstanding illnesses and disabilities (Briggs 1993), but dementia probably puts the most stress on a sufferer's support network (Gilleard 1984). The availability and adaptability of support networks are important determinants of the need for community health and social services and residential care (Wenger and Shahtamasebi 1990; Scott and Wenger 1994). Thus it is important to understand how support networks change as people get older and their circumstances change, and the extent to which this change is gendered.

In this chapter, we describe the influences affecting the development of support networks for men and women and introduce five types of support networks identified during a longitudinal study in North Wales. We describe how network type is related to gender, marital status and parenthood and discuss the implications of network type for informal support in old age.

The development of support networks

Each person's support network is part of a larger social network consisting of family, friends and neighbours (Wenger 1984). The size and constitution of these networks depend to a great extent on demographic factors such as marriage, fertility and mortality as well as migration behaviour of the individual and of others in the network.

Family

The basis of most people's support network is the family. The numbers of children one's parents and grandparents had determines the presence of sisters, brothers, aunts and uncles. Their fertility in turn affects the numbers of nephews, nieces and cousins. As people age, same-generation relatives are increasingly lost from the support network by death. Since women live longer than men (Coleman *et al.* 1993), they are more likely than men to outlive their siblings. Thus women tend to have fewer brothers and sisters in old age, and both men and women are more likely to have sisters than brothers.

Marriage increases the number of relatives by including in-laws and gives the potential for further expansion with children and grandchildren. However, marriage patterns are affected by the availability of suitable partners at the appropriate stage of life. For those who grew up in the first half of the twentieth century, the effect of the two world wars was to reduce the numbers of men of marriageable age, so that women were more likely than men to remain single or to be widowed before completing a family.

Spouses have been shown to be the most important source of companionship, intimate closeness and well-being (Quinn *et al.* 1984) and being married is highly associated with contentment in old age (Hunt 1978). However, there are indications that marriage is more beneficial for older men than for older women. Married women suffer higher rates of depression (Gove and Tudor 1973) and higher rates of loneliness than married men (Wenger 1983), although the latter is likely to be rationalized or concealed.

Although marriage has the potential to increase support network size, Wenger (1984) found this varied with marital status only for men. Single and widowed women had support networks of similar size to married women, but single men tended to have smaller networks and the support networks of married men tended to shrink if they were widowed (Wenger 1986).

Married or widowed people tend to concentrate demands for help on one person while those who have never married, or are childless, are more likely to spread their needs throughout their networks. Thus, even though the number of people available may be larger, the composition of the support network may depend more on the types of relationships involved. Married men are more likely than women to develop relationships through their spouses or to depend on their spouse's relationships with others (Wenger 1992b), but if they are widowed these networks contract. Single women tend to have larger support networks than single men but, for both genders, the absence of a spouse and/or adult children means that there is no one in the network for whom normative expectations of care in old age exist (Wenger 1992b). Single women's larger networks provide more expressive support but single men can become quite isolated.

The differing life expectancies of men and women in middle and old age also affect patterns of marital status. Shorter life expectancy for men and the tendency of men to marry women younger than themselves means that they are more likely to remain married whereas elderly women are more likely to be widowed. In addition, widowed men are more likely to remarry. This is partly because men have a greater number of potential partners available (because of the greater longevity of women), as well as cultural expectations that support men marrying much younger wives, but older men also seem more inclined to remarry when they find a suitable potential partner than do older women (see Gail Wilson's Chapter 8).

Although widowhood entails the loss of the person who is most often the central figure in the support network, it does not necessarily result in a decrease in network size. Sisters-in-law and brothers-in-law often remain close to their sibling's widowed spouse in much the same way as blood relatives do (Wenger 1992b). If the bereavement has been preceded by a period of caring for the spouse during their final illness, the release from this responsibility may allow for an increase in social activity, although it is usually easier for widows than widowers to re-establish a social life and join the society of other widows and voluntary organizations. It is more difficult for widowed men for a number of reasons. First, mutual support between widowers is not often available or culturally accepted as a norm. Second, men who become spouse carers tend to do so at greater ages than women and to care for longer periods (Wenger 1990); as a result they are older, less well and less able to resume or re-establish a social life after widowhood. Third, the members of men's support networks tend to be the associates of their wives and they are likely to have fewer friends (of either gender) in their networks than women.

Widows and widowers often move to be closer to their adult children, in anticipation of, or as a result of, increasing age and frailty. These changes can result in a change in network type (see below). Widowed women tend to maintain larger networks than do widowed men, as noted above (Wenger 1984; Mugford and Kendig 1986).

The main difference in family patterns between men and women as they age is the greater proportion of women who are widowed, and this difference increases for those in the oldest age groups. However, amongst the present elderly cohorts, women are also less likely than men to have ever married. Older women have fewer close relatives of all kinds than older men and are more likely than men to live alone in old age.

Friends and neighbours

It has been suggested that good friends and neighbours are more important than family in old age (Abrams 1978). While the networks of both men and women are family based, women's networks tend to have more extra-familial bonds (Corin 1982). Older men's networks tend to be more focused on their children (where they have them) and on their own neighbourhood.

The importance of friendship in later life has been well-documented (Francis 1984; Wenger 1987a; Jerrome 1993). Women are more likely than men to have (and maintain) close confiding relationships with same-sex friends (Lowenthal and Robinson 1976; Mugford and Kendig 1986; Jerrome 1990), although this too is influenced by life expectancy. Very old men often feel isolated from peers; particularly in a rural setting they can become the sole male survivor in their local age group.

Long-standing same-sex friendships are especially important (Francis 1984) and the sources of such friendships differ for men and women. While both genders may retain friendships from their schooldays, men's subsequent friendships have been mainly related to work or leisure activities. The genesis of women's friendships, on the other hand, tends to be associated with shared neighbourhood and shared life stage experiences such as marriage, child-bearing and childraising. Their friendships are, therefore, less likely to be affected by ageing and retirement than are men's friendships. Women continue to share the experience of marriage or widowhood and the centrality of family life.

There are, however, interesting rural–urban differences in friendship vis-à-vis gender. In rural areas women tend to move into their husband's community on marriage (Wenger 1980), while in urban areas preferred residence has been near to the wife's mother so that husbands are more likely to move into the wife's neighbourhood (Rosser and Harris 1965). Women in rural areas may, therefore, be expected to be more dependent on friendship than their urban sisters, although urban women (in the absence of migration) may be more integrated into their localities (Wenger 1995). On the other hand, rural men are more likely to retain local ties in rural areas, although in both contexts women are more likely to have same-sex friends than men. Men are less likely than women to visit friends (Wenger 1984). Bayley *et al.* (1982) found that two-thirds of all visits to older people were from women.

Friendship needs change over the life course and there are clear gender differences (Wenger 1987a; Jerrome 1990). Men's friendships continue to be based on shared activities and sociability while women's friendships are more intimate and intense and tend to focus on conversation and mutual support. Friendship for women continues to be meaningful and often extensive well into old age (Jerrome 1990). Women talk about their friendships more than men do (Wenger 1987a). Older men talk less about their friendships and give the impression that these relationships are less close than those between women. Most interaction between men takes place outside the home, whereas women visit one another's homes. There is less evidence of mutual support between men, although cross-sex support (men supporting women and women supporting men) appears to be more likely (Wenger 1987a).

Women tend to continue to make new friends throughout the life course, whereas men are less likely to replace lost friendships. As a result it has been suggested that women have a psychological advantage (Myerhoff 1978). But women and working-class older people lose friends more often than men and middle-class people due to the greater average age of women and the higher mortality rates of the working class. One study has found that women are more likely than men to wish for more friends (Wenger 1987a); this is probably not unrelated to their capacity to make new friends.

The increased leisure time of the postretirement years means more opportunity for involvement in voluntary groups. Generally, women tend to be more involved with community organizations than men in rural areas (Wenger 1984), but there is some indication that men are more involved in urban areas (Hunt 1978). There are also distinct social class differences (Jerrome 1990; Wenger 1992b). Both men and women with middle-class status tend to be involved in age-mixed voluntary groups and other aspects of public life. Working-class men also have a tradition of group membership (Jerrome 1990), although this is likely to be more pronounced in urban areas. However, involvement in voluntary groups decreases with advancing age (Wenger 1984). Old people's clubs are primarily attractive to working-class people and members of all clubs usually attend with friends (Wenger 1987a; Jerrome 1990). Older men sometimes do not wish to become involved with old people's organizations which they see as dominated by women, as discussed by Wilson (Chapter 8)

Social class and migration

Social class has an effect on networks as a result of differential resources and geographical mobility. Middle-class people are more likely to migrate at all stages of life. Moves before retirement age are usually associated with employment, whereas later moves are primarily to live in a more desirable area or to be near relatives. Retirement migrants are usually married couples. An individual's network is affected not only by their own moves, but by the movement of other network members. Although the present generation of elderly people has a low level of migration, their children and grandchildren are increasingly mobile.

While middle-class networks are more likely to be widely dispersed, they are less likely to be constrained by distance because they have greater access to transport and telephones (d'Abbs 1982). Middle-class networks are also more heterogeneous and include more friends. Middle-class people are more likely to make a distinction between friends and neighbours and to turn to friends, rather than family, for help (Warren 1981).

Older working-class people, on the other hand, have smaller social networks (Corin 1982), which are kin-dominated, the mother–daughter link being especially strong in western societies (d'Abbs 1982), and are often based on longstanding residence in the same community. The numerical predominance of women in the elderly population is more marked among the working class, because the relationship between life expectancy and social class is stronger for men than for women (Arber and Ginn 1993b). Working-class men are more likely to die before retirement and to die at younger ages after retirement. Older women, therefore, are more likely to come from working-class backgrounds than are older men.

Health

Men, despite lower life expectancy, experience better health than women do in old age (Arber and Ginn 1991a), and on average have shorter terminal illnesses. Women, on the other hand, are more subject to the degenerative diseases of advanced old age. Women live longer in poor health while older men are less likely to be limited by physical disability than women (Wenger 1987b). The *active life expectancy* (the number of years a person can expect to survive without significant disability) is not much greater for women than for men, despite women's greater total life expectancy (Arber and Ginn 1991a).

Poor health does not seem to be associated with reduction in average size of support network for those who remain living in the community. For the majority of very elderly people, network size increases as relatives become more involved in providing care. However, a minority of older people are affected by social isolation (lack of contact with others), and this tends to increase with failing health (Wenger 1984). For these people, network members may be less aware of the need for help.

Personal care in illness and disability is provided by close relatives, most commonly a spouse, or an adult child (Wenger 1987b). Because of the greater likelihood of being widowed for women and the strong attachments between mothers and daughters, men are more likely to be cared for by wives and women by daughters. This means that elderly men are more likely to be tended by elderly women and elderly women by middle aged women, although with increasing numbers of people living into their 90s, a caring son or daughter may themselves be over retirement age.

When an older person needs personal care and has no close relatives, they have to rely on care which is privately purchased or provided by the state. This often means residential care, and women are much more likely than men to be in residential care in later life (Arber and Ginn 1991a).

Support network types

A typology of support networks has been developed, based initially on a longitudinal study of ageing conducted in North Wales from 1979–91 (Wenger 1984, 1986). Survey interviews were conducted with 534 people aged 65 and over and living at home in 1979, and follow-up surveys of survivors were conducted in 1983, 1987 and 1991. In addition, an intensive study of 30 people aged 79 and over was conducted from 1983–87 which provided qualitative data to support the quantitative data from the survey interviews. The original study used an adaptation of the methodology developed by McAllister and Fischer (1978), described in Wenger (1984).

The North Wales study, in a primarily rural area, resulted in the identification of five different types of support networks based on: (1) the availability of local close kin; (2) the level of involvement of family, friends and neighbours, and (3) the level of interaction with the community and voluntary groups.

The networks are named on the basis of the nature of the older person's relationship to the support network. The first three types are based on the presence of local kin, while the other two types reflect the absence of local kin. The five network types identified can be summarized as follows:

1 *The local family dependent support network* has its primary focus on close local family ties, with few peripheral friends and neighbours. It is often based on a shared household with, or near to, an adult child, often a daughter. Community involvement is generally low. All support needs are met by relatives. These networks tend to be small and the people are more likely to be widowed, older and in less good health than those with other types of networks.

2 *The locally integrated support network* includes close relationships with local family, friends and neighbours. Many neighbours are also friends. Usually based on long term residence and active community involvement in church and voluntary organizations in the present or recent past, these networks tend to be larger on average than others.

3 *The local self-contained support network* typically has arm's length relationships or infrequent contact with at least one relative living in the same or adjacent

community or neighbourhood, often a sibling, niece or nephew. Childlessness is common. Reliance is mainly on neighbours but elderly people with this type of network tend to adopt a household focused lifestyle and community involvement, if any, tends to be low. Networks tend to be smaller than average.

4 *The wider community focused network* is associated with active relationships with distant relatives, usually children, and high salience of friends and neighbours. Absence of local kin is typical. The distinction between friends and neighbours is maintained. The people are generally involved in community and/or voluntary organizations. This type of network is frequently associated with retirement migration and is commonly a middle-class or skilled working-class adaptation. Networks are larger than average.

5 *The private restricted support network* is typically associated with absence of local kin, other than in some cases a spouse, although a high proportion are married. Contact with neighbours is minimal. These people have few nearby friends and a low level of community contacts or involvements. The network type subsumes two subtypes: independent married couples and dependent persons who have withdrawn or become isolated from local involvement. In many cases a low level of social contact represents a lifelong adaptation. Networks are smaller than average.

The network typology was subsequently operationalized as a survey instrument and further studies with rural and urban populations have demonstrated its generalizability to other settings. In this chapter we present comparative data from the North Wales Longitudinal Study 1979 survey and from ALPHA, an epidemiological survey in Liverpool concerned primarily with the incidence of dementia (Wenger 1995). The latter study involved a sample of 5,222 people aged 65 and over, stratified by age and sex, living in the community or in residential care. During the first wave of interviews in 1989–91, network type was determined for 4,496 respondents living in the community.

The distribution of network types

The distribution of network types is related to a wide range of demographic and social variables (Wenger and Shahtamasebi 1990; Wenger 1995). Table 12.1 shows the distribution of network types in the population aged 65 and over for men, women and all respondents in North Wales and in Liverpool. These estimates have been obtained by weighting the stratified samples to match the populations from which they were drawn. Although there are some similarities, there are significant differences between the overall distributions for North Wales and Liverpool, as well as gender differences that manifest themselves differently in the two settings.

Table 12.1   Proportion of men and women aged 65+ in each network type in North Wales (1979) and Liverpool (1989–91)

Network type	North Wales			Liverpool		
	Men %	Women %	All %	Men %	Women %	All %
Family dependent	23	23	23	23	23	23
Locally integrated	35	29	32	44	49	47
Local self-contained	14	22	19	13	11	12
Wider community focused	17	16	17	4	5	5
Private restricted	11	10	10	16	12	13
N =	204	321	525	2179	2317	4496

Note: Percentages are weighted to adjust for stratification of samples, and do not always add up to 100 per cent because of rounding.

The commonest network type is the *locally integrated*, which comprised one-third of networks in North Wales and nearly half in Liverpool. This is followed by *local family dependent*, at just under a quarter of networks in both areas. The third type involving local kin, *locally self-contained* networks, formed nearly a fifth of the North Wales networks, and was less common in Liverpool. However, the total with local kin was higher in Liverpool at 82 per cent, compared with 73 per cent in North Wales.

Among those without local kin, the *wider community focused* type was common in North Wales, at 17 per cent, mainly because of retired migrants. However, this type was rare in Liverpool's stable working-class elderly community, at only 5 per cent, whereas the *private restricted* type was somewhat more common (13 per cent compared to 10 per cent).

The distribution of network types found in a cross-sectional study is the result of a number of interacting factors, which operate differently for men and women and in different types of community. Networks tend to shift as people get older and more dependent, but people who are dependent are also those most likely to die or enter residential care, so that there is some stability in network distribution as the population remaining in the community gets older. However, entry into residential care is less likely when there are relatives who can care for the older person at home. Women live longer and are more prone to disability in old age than men, but they are also less likely to have close relatives to care for them and more likely to go into residential care. The availability of nearby relatives also varies between types of community. When the population is denser and more stable, as in Liverpool, more relatives, friends and neighbours are likely to be available for inclusion in the support network, and this explains the higher prevalence of locally integrated networks in Liverpool, compared to North Wales, where the population is sparse and even 'local' migration can involve relatively large separations in terms of geographical distance and transport.

The remainder of this section concerns the way ageing, marriage and parenthood affect men's and women's networks.

Network changes during later life

Longitudinal analysis in the North Wales study has shown that support network type can change with the passage of time, and that predictable shifts occur in the face of changes in dependency and of certain types of relationships (Wenger 1992b). Figure 12.1 shows the percentage of networks of each type that shifted to each destination type, when all opportunities for shift (that is, two consecutive assessments of network type during the four phases in 1979, 1983, 1987 and 1991) were pooled.

In interpreting these patterns of network shifts, it should be borne in mind that respondents who died or moved into residential care, or were not followed up for other reasons, are not included in the totals for calculating percentages. Thus, the family dependent network type is the least likely to change between assessments (80 per cent remaining the same), but this type also includes more of the very old and most dependent respondents than other types, so it may not be the most stable type when shifts to residential care are also included. Certain shifts in network type are more likely than others. Shifts in both directions between *family dependent* and *locally integrated* types were common, as were those between *wider community focused* and *private restricted* types. However, *local self-contained* types were most likely to shift *to* either family dependent or private restricted networks. The local self-contained type was less common as a destination type; when it was, the shift was likely to be *from* locally integrated or private restricted.

Particular shifts in network type are often associated with specific changes in circumstances. As health deteriorates, locally integrated networks tend to become family dependent if close relatives are available, but may also become local self-contained, when neighbours assume support roles, as long as personal care is not required. Wider community focused networks, where there are no local family members apart perhaps from a spouse, tend to change to private restricted, as friends die or move into residential care and activities are restricted through loss of mobility. Private restricted networks are the least able to adapt to increased dependency. People with these networks are the most likely to depend on formal services and to enter residential care.

There are a smaller number of changes in the opposite direction, from family dependent to locally integrated or private restricted to wider community focused, and these are usually associated with an improvement in health or release from caring responsibilities.

Network shifts are sometimes associated with the death of a spouse, but the nature of such shifts varies. The initial reaction to bereavement might be withdrawal from community contacts to a family dependent network, perhaps

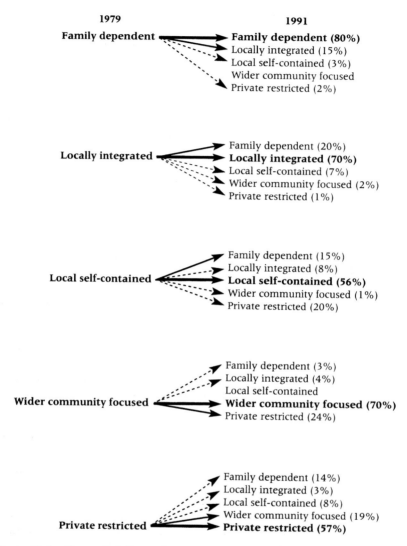

Figure 12.1   Network shifts in the North Wales longitudinal study 1979–91

accompanied by a move to be nearer family. If there are no nearby family members, the network is likely to become private restricted. However, shifts are also observed in the opposite direction following the bereavement period, with increased community involvement, particularly among women.

The result of these shifts is that with advancing age people are more likely to have local family dependent or private restricted network types and less likely to have locally integrated or wider community focused networks. This is true for men and women, so it might be expected that women, being older and likely to have poorer health, would be concentrated more in the dependent network types (family dependent and private restricted). However, this is not borne out in the distributions shown in Table 12.1. In the North Wales study (although the numbers are not large enough for the differences to be statistically significant) there was a higher proportion of women in local self-contained networks. It is likely that women's traditional roles are more conducive to the household-focused lifestyle associated with this network type.

The results from Liverpool are different from those expected, with significantly more women than men in locally integrated networks (which are more frequent in the younger age groups) and significantly more men than women in private restricted networks (which are more frequent in the older age groups). The Liverpool sample has not been studied for long enough to observe network shifts in the long term, but the relationship between network type and age in the baseline survey was similar to that in North Wales.

A partial explanation for these anomalies is that among those who would otherwise be in the dependent network types, women are more likely to be in residential care. However, other factors also play a part; women tend to have more friends, to be involved more in community activities, and to adapt better to widowhood than men of the same age.

Further analysis of the Liverpool data using multivariate techniques, and use of the network typology in other settings, may lead to a greater understanding of the relative importance of these factors in determining the network types of men and women. Analysis of data from the first phase of the North Wales longitudinal study has shown statistically significant differences in the effects of marriage and parenthood for men and women, which we describe below.

Marriage and parenthood

A large majority of people marry and most of those who marry become parents. The minority of elderly people who have never married, and those who have married but not had children, show differences in support network type compared with the majority. People who marry acquire more relatives and their spouse's friends may also become available as support network members. This does not mean, however, that husbands and wives always have the same support network type; their support network types may have different membership and/or frequency of contacts.

In the North Wales study, the locally integrated type was less common for people who had never been married, and both single men and single women were most likely to have local self-contained support networks (characterized as household-centred with primary reliance on neighbours), with locally integrated networks coming a close second. For single women, the wider community focused network type (based on friendship and membership of voluntary organizations) was more common than average, but this type was hardly seen among single men, who were more likely to adopt a privatized lifestyle.

For women, motherhood made the family dependent network type as common as the locally integrated one. Childless women who were, or had been, married, had similar network types to single women, with local self-contained the commonest type. These women were also more likely than mothers to have private restricted network types.

Widows formed a majority of the women in the sample, but widowhood was not reflected in reduced contact with kin. Although the numbers were small, childless widows showed the same pattern of contact with kin as childless married women. It was motherhood that made a difference. Thus having children, for women, appears to be critical in terms of the nature of support in old age.

In contrast, fatherhood made no significant difference to network type; the networks of fathers and childless married men were similar. The only difference was an increase in private restricted types for childless men (which was not, however, statistically significant). This was confined to currently-married men and reflects the couple centred private lifestyle of many childless couples. This network type was not found among the few childless widowers.

Men are less likely to be widowed in old age than women and so are less likely to depend on children in old age. Their best insurance for a well-supported old age is marriage, rather than parenthood. Perhaps this explains the greater desire for remarriage amongst widowed men (see Wilson's Chapter 8).

Sources of support within networks

Differences in marital status between older men and women not only affect network type but also the *source* and *nature* of support. For most married people their spouse is the main source of support. The normative expectations of help from spouses are for 'total help, support and personal care as needed' unless the spouse is in poor mental or physical health (Wenger 1994b: 12).

Most older men receive their main support from wives living in the same household. Most older women are widowed and about half receive their main support from adult children, most of whom are living in other households at various distances from their mother's home. The normative expectations of help from children are for 'frequent contact, moral support, problem solving, emergency help, regular help where needed and inclusion in family occasions' (Wenger 1994b: 12). These expectations are affected by distance, gender and marital status of the adult child.

Widowed fathers also rely on adult children. For all men and women in the North Wales study, reliance on children was more common the more children they had. However, while just over half of widowed parents relied on children, the remainder tended to say that they relied primarily on themselves or on no one.

Single and widowed people without children, if they were not self-reliant, were most likely to rely on another relative (sister, brother, niece or nephew), with single people of both genders more likely to rely on a sister or brother. Similar proportions of men and women relied most on a friend or neighbour, when there were no spouse or children. Overall, women were more likely than men to say they were self-reliant, even when those who relied on their spouse or adult children were excluded.

Implications for caring

Because more older men are married, help is likely to be more immediately available than for older women and thus better able to deal with short-interval or unpredictable needs within the context of an intimate relationship. However, their wives are also older and more often in less than good health than adult child carers. Help for older women, on the other hand, comes mainly from younger generation helpers living in other households. Predictable needs can be routinized but help for unpredictable needs or emergencies must be summoned from a distance. Adult children are usually in better health and more likely to drive than older wives, but they also have conflicting work and family responsibilities. Arguably, therefore, older men receive more available and predictable supportive help than older women do. Although the support older women receive from younger family members tends to be less immediately available, these helpers may provide pathways to a wider range of resources.

So far, we have looked at support from the point of view of the recipient. Older people also give support. Although women are more likely than men to be widowed, their spouses are more likely to die suddenly, whereas men whose wives die are more likely to have nursed them during a prolonged terminal illness (Wenger 1990). If they live into their 80s, the likelihood of caring for a dependent spouse is almost as great for men as for women. Husbands who provide care are older than wives who do so, and they tend to care for longer.

The nature of caring between older spouses is discussed by Rose and Bruce (Chapter 9). Traditional differences in tasks considered appropriate to men and women are frequently abandoned in the face of necessity, but husbands are more likely to delegate intimate care to another relative where possible. Evidence from the North Wales study suggests that older husbands rely primarily on their wives for both expressive and instrumental help, whereas older wives tend to look outside marriage for significant proportions of emotional support.

Conclusions

Patterns of support in old age result from a complex interaction of social and demographic factors. The type and nature of informal support available depends on the individual's type of support network. Three major factors influence the formation of support networks: marriage and fertility patterns (of the individual and of their parents' and grandparents' generations); migration history (of the individual, their family and of the community in which they live); and personality. The individual may have little control over most of these factors. Personality affects the nature of our relationships with those around us, but its effect on the size and composition of our support network is limited by the availability of potential network members. The most significant factor – the marriage and fertility patterns of earlier generations – is beyond the control of the individual. Our own history, in terms of the childbearing of our parents and grandparents, therefore, makes an important contribution to the type of help that will be available in old age. The impact of this is no different for men or women.

As a result of women's greater life expectancy and the age differential in marriage, most men can expect to be supported by wives in old age while most women rely on help from another source. There are indications that most unmarried older people prefer to be independent and self-reliant. However, in the face of advanced age and/or physical impairment, parenthood is more important for the support of older women than for men because of women's greater likelihood of widowhood.

The shorter life expectancy of men, paradoxically, appears to act in their favour. They tend to experience shorter periods of incapacity before death, and are less likely to be widowed and to face adaptation to living alone. Because their wives generally outlive them they can anticipate care and support in their old age, whether or not they have children. Men, therefore, are less likely to become reliant on their children and are less affected by the childbearing of their parents and grandparents. Those men who have never married, however, are disadvantaged. Also, when men become carers themselves in old age, they are likely be older and to care for longer than women do.

Women, on the other hand, are likely to suffer from more severe mobility problems or longer periods of terminal illness, to be widowed, to live alone and to depend on the support of their children. Parenthood is, therefore, more important as a source of social, practical and emotional support for older women and those who are childless are disadvantaged.

Our elderly population is dominated by women, particularly widows. The widow has a much more established role in society that the widower. Women who have spent much of their adult life in childrearing and other home-based activities have more opportunity to develop the types of social relationships that can continue into the retirement years. On the other hand, men whose social life in middle age is centred around work and leisure activities may have difficulty in adapting to a home and neighbourhood focused lifestyle when those activities are no longer possible. Women who suffer bereavement and incapacity are more likely than men to have peers in the same situation. Perhaps because of the existence of these role models, women seem more able to cope with the losses and problems that they are more likely to suffer in old age.

CONNECTING GENDER AND AGEING: A NEW BEGINNING?

Sara Arber and Jay Ginn

The chapters in this volume have shown that by connecting gender and ageing both the sociology of gender and the sociology of ageing are strengthened; the reworking of theoretical ideas within both subdisciplines spills over to enrich mainstream sociology. A key issue is to what extent ageing represents liberation from rigid gender role expectations and an opportunity for women to be independent and self-determining, and for men to take on new roles and ways of relating to others.

This volume has begun the task of exploring the relationship between ageing and gender, focusing both on the private and public domain. Hitherto, little sociological attention has been devoted to men's role in the private domain following their exit from paid employment, and the negotiation of new gender roles and relationships.

Later life continues to straddle the public and private worlds, but in ways that vary for older women and men, and according to class, race and ethnicity. Consumption and lifestyles are important orienting concerns for older people, but are themselves affected by previous roles in the productive and reproductive spheres. An emphasis in this volume has been to hear the voices of older people themselves, letting them define issues of concern rather than imposing the ageist concerns of social scientists; for too long older people have been conceptualized as a burden on society and family members, primarily studied in terms of a range of social problems, from poverty to ill-health and disability.

To make theoretical progress, there is a need to clarify the various meanings of ageing and how they are gendered. Gender is inextricably bound up with different meanings of ageing, which are related, yet conceptually distinct. Chronological age is a marker for transitions of status in our society, as well as access to rights and benefits. For most of the twentieth century, the age of eligibility for the British state pension has been five years lower for women than men, which may have reinforced the widespread prejudice that women 'age' earlier than men, becoming unfit for work in their 50s.

Physiological ageing differs for women and men; women aged over 65 are more likely than men to experience chronic illnesses which restrict mobility and their capacity to live independently of assistance from family members, non-kin or the state. Thus although women's life expectancy is over five years longer than men's, the gender gap in expectation of disability-free years (active life expectancy) is much narrower. This gender difference in physiological ageing, coupled with the age differential in marriage, means that women are more likely to be widowed than men, and are more reliant on wider kin networks and the state for assistance, as discussed in Chapter 12.

The social meaning of age is profoundly gendered. The 'double standard of ageing', in which women but not men are expected to retain a youthful appearance, warding off the signs of ageing for as long as possible, is widely recognized. McDaniel (1988: 16) sums this up by quoting Oscar Wilde: 'A man's face is his autobiography, a woman's her greatest work of fiction'. Chapter 5 shows how gendered ageism by employers affects women's opportunities for employment and promotion, a practice which increasingly hampers women's efforts to find and keep a job after age 55.

Despite the combined effects of ageism and sexism in cultural attitudes towards older women, the chapters in this book demonstrate how older women may be developing a more authentic identity and orientation, especially following widowhood, when they are no longer constrained to fulfil gendered role obligations expected within marriage. Chapter 8 shows that older widows are likely to reject the idea of remarriage, which is seen as having few benefits for older women and a range of disadvantages. Chapter 4 illustrates alternative ways in which women's conflicts between their desire to conform to prescribed gender roles and their desire for autonomy can be resolved in later life, while also showing the importance of continuity of aspects of gender role identity over time.

Among older married couples, gender role identity becomes more fluid, for example, the performance of previously gender-related tasks may become more interchangeable between women and men, in response to the functional disability of either partner. Chapters 8 and 9 demonstrate couples' determination to maintain their independence, which tends to override previous gendered roles. However, analysis of the meaning and language of caring (in Chapter 9) demonstrates the subtle ways in which gendered power relationships and gender-differentiated esteem may persist, despite ostensible gender equivalence in the performance of domestic and caring tasks.

The study of ageing must embrace a dynamic perspective in two senses. First, the individual's previous biography, in terms of both family and work roles, has a profound influence on their resources, roles and relationships in later life. Second, living through particular secular (or period) changes at different stages of the life course affects individuals' attitudes towards gender roles. The current generation of older people span a wide range of birth cohorts, those who grew up before World War I lived through different experiences from those who were children during the interwar depression. As Mannheim (1952) reminds us, the social norms and attitudes extant in our formative years continue to influence behaviour and attitudes throughout the life course. The next generation of older people who grew up in the 1950s and 1960s will have been affected by second wave feminism and are likely to enter later life with very different employment experiences and gender role expectations.

A full understanding of gender and ageing requires the merging of the micro perspective, of gender roles and relationships, with the macro perspective, which takes account of wider societal changes, as advocated in Chapter 2. Such macro-level changes have had major effects on the lives of older women and men. For example the progressively earlier age of exit from paid employment and improving health of the population have meant that women and men spend many more active years without paid work both before and after the state pension age than in the past. More importantly, state provision in the form of the National Insurance retirement pension, has made it possible for older people to live independently of both paid work and of financial support from a spouse or other relatives, a situation which is unprecedented historically (Wall 1992). However, it is important to consider trends in social and economic policy which threaten to reverse these gains, particularly for older women. Although older women have always been poorer than older men, the state National Insurance pension has meant that since the 1950s older women have had more independent financial resources than in the past, promoting their opportunities for independent action and social citizenship. However, the signs are that these opportunities are under threat.

As Walby (1994) argues, women do not have the same access to citizenship as men, particularly in relation to 'civil' and 'social' rights. Civil rights include the rights to bodily integrity, not to be beaten by a partner or carer, and the right to work at the occupation of the individual's choice. The rights of social citizenship are bound up both with being a worker, and with the welfare state 'provision of an infrastructure which enables people to be guaranteed a minimum provision of necessities' (1994: 389). We need to consider how ageing and gender intersect in terms of differential access to citizenship. Since historically citizenship has been linked to participation in the public sphere, it is perhaps unsurprising that British older women lack full access to the rights of social and civil citizenship.

British government policies since 1979 have emphasized an ideology of individualism and self-provision, rather than state responsibility, for example, promoting private pensions through incentives, while allowing the value of the state basic pension to fall. Although such policies are presented as gender-neutral, they are inherently gendered in their assumptions and consequences. The state pension has declined in real value since 1980 when indexing to average earnings was replaced by indexing to prices; it is projected to decline to only 10 per cent of male earnings by 2020 (Evandrou and Falkingham 1993), and is falling increasingly far below the means-tested Income Support level. Since the majority of older women have no other source of independent income than the state pension (Ginn and Arber 1991, 1994a), their income is below the level of means-tested benefits, leaving them, by definition, in poverty.

The British government has argued that the state pension is of diminishing importance because two-thirds of the recently retired have independent (mainly occupational) pensions. For example, the government-appointed Social Security Advisory Committee (1992: 12) stated: 'Now almost two-thirds of those who retire can do so with an occupational pension' and the Secretary of State for Social Security has continued to propagate the myth that a majority of older people have an occupational pension: 'nearly 70 per cent of those now retiring . . . will have supplemented their income in this way' (Lilley 1992: 8). Such statements are widely quoted by the media, but are misleading because they ignore married women, counting them as receiving their husbands' pensions. In fact less than half of people aged 55 to 69 have entitlement to an occupational pension, but this is 68 per cent of men and only 29 per cent of women (Bone *et al.* 1992: Table 6.1). Older married women are therefore invisible in the government's portrayal of pensioners' sources of income. There is no acknowledgement that the majority of women will be widowed and that provision of widows' benefits in occupational pension schemes is patchy and inadequate. The greater the movement towards individual provision for retirement through occupational and personal pensions as the major source of income in later life, the greater will be the income inequality between older women and men, and between those who have had an intermittent or low paid employment history and those with an advantaged position in the labour market. Thus the opportunities to enjoy a Third Age of self-development and autonomous action are likely to become increasingly gendered, as well as class-divided, with financial dependency acting as an obstacle to citizenship rights.

Government plans to raise women's state pension age to 65 from the year 2010 will exacerbate women's disadvantage, by widening the gap between their last employment and the age when they can claim state pensions. Although presented as progressive legislation to ensure equal treatment of men and women, this proposal ignores gendered ageism in the labour market, which results in women being considered 'too old' for a job at an earlier age than men (Chapter 5), as well as the handicaps faced by women in obtaining occupational pensions. Because of these gendered processes in employment, raising women's state pension age will leave married women without an income of their own for a number of years, while non-married women may be forced to rely on Income Support.

Another major social policy change affecting older people is access to state-provided health and domiciliary care. The Community Care Act was implemented in 1993, ostensibly based on a rationale of independence and choice for the older person, but the reality is that 'social' care is less likely to be provided by the state than in the past. Hospitals are increasingly discharging older patients who in the past would have received continuing nursing care, so that relatives are required to provide care. Older people who lack available relatives to provide care are obliged to pay for social care, whether this is provided at home or in a residential establishment. All these changes have gendered consequences, disadvantaging older women to a far greater extent than older men. As discussed in Chapter 12, older men are more likely to have wives to rely on to provide care should they need it, but older women are more likely to be widowed and reliant on wider kin and the state.

It is well known that women are more likely than men to provide informal care for older relatives, and therefore any curtailing of state provision has a greater adverse effect on women both as care-receivers and as carers (Kaden and McDaniel 1990). What is less well known is that women employees are more likely to suffer adverse job and career effects because of providing care than equivalent men carers, as shown in Chapter 10. The increasing reliance of older women on adult children and wider kin for informal care may result in more older women suffering 'elder abuse'. Chapter 11 provides a convincing analysis of the ways in which current research and theorizing about elder abuse obscures the gendered nature of such abuse.

Many other macro-level societal and legislative changes have differential impacts on older women and men, reducing the opportunities for older women to live full and autonomous lives. For example, reductions in public transport, the increase in out-of-town shopping areas, increases in crime and fears about crime and safety all have worse consequences for older women than men. Reducing the role of the welfare state is also occurring in other western countries. Our view accords with that of Hendricks and Rosenthal (1993: 3): 'while social structure may limit possibilities, daily lives must be seen in terms of individual intentionality. The goal is an understanding of how individual actors create the connections between individual and structural facets of their identity'.

Despite the scenario for the future looking bleak at the macro level, this volume has shown that older women have considerable social resources, particularly relating to their wider friendship networks and closer emotional relationships with others. Their earlier lives may have equipped older women with a better ability than men to cope with many of the privations of later life.

Ageing potentially liberates older women from the restrictions placed upon them by their family, conventional gender roles and their portrayal by others as sex-objects. We end on an optimistic note:

Three sets of factors intertwine to make the role of older women increasingly important in the future. First is our growing numerical strength with its potential political power. Second is the struggles experienced by many older women against poverty, institutionalization, and the combined effects of ageism and sexism. Third is the gender-structured positions held by women in our society which teach us to care and connect with others in both perception and action.

(McDaniel 1988: 22)

REFERENCES

Abbott, P. and Wallace, C. (1990) *An Introduction to Sociology: Feminist Perspectives*. London: Routledge.

Abdela, L. (1991) *Breaking Through Glass Ceilings: A Practical Guide to Equality at Work for Women and Men*. Solihull: METRA.

Abdela, R. S. (1984) *Equality in Employment*, A Royal Commission Report, Ottawa: Ministry of Supply and Services.

Abrams, M. (1978) *Beyond Three-Score and Ten: A First Report on a Survey of the Elderly*. Mitchum, Surrey: Age Concern.

Abrams, P., Abrams, S., Humprey, R. and Snaith, R. (1989) *Neighbourhood Care and Social Policy*. London: HMSO.

Abu-Laban, S. M. (1981) Women and aging: A futuristic perspective, *Psychology of Women Quarterly*, 6: 85–98.

Acker, J. (1980) Women and stratification: A review of recent literature, *Contemporary Sociology*, 9: 25–34.

Acker, J. (1988) Class, gender and the relations of distribution, *Signs*, 13(8): 473–97.

Ade-Ridder, L. (1990) Sexuality and marital quality among older married couples. In T. Brubaker (ed.) *Family Relationships in Later Life*, 2nd edn. London: Sage.

Allatt, P., Keil, T., Bryman, A. and Bytheway B. (eds) (1987) *Women and the Life Cycle: Transitions and Turning Points*. London: Macmillan.

Anderson, A. and Ingrisch, D. (1992) *Untersuchung zu gesellschaftlichen Leitbildern und individuellen Wirklichkeiten im Alterungsprozeß von Frauen*, unpublished research report. Vienna.

Anderson, M. (1983) *Thinking About Women – Sociological and Feminist Perspectives*. New York: Macmillan.

Anderson, S., Russell, C. and Schumm, W. (1983) Perceived marital quality and family life-cycle categories: A further analysis, *Journal of Marriage and the Family*, 45: 127–39.

Arber, S. (1989) Class and the elderly, *Social Studies Review*, 4(3): 90–95.

Arber, S. and Evandrou, M. (eds) (1993) *Ageing, Independence and the Life Course*. London: Jessica Kingsley Publishers.

Arber, S. and Gilbert, G.N. (1989a) Men: The forgotten carers, *Sociology* 23 (1): 111–18.

Arber, S. and Gilbert, G. N. (1989b) Transitions in caring: Gender, life course and the care of the elderly. In B. Bytheway, T. Keil, P. Allatt and A. Bryman (eds) *Becoming and Being Old: Sociological Approaches to Later Life*. London: Sage.

Arber, S. and Ginn, J. (1990) The meaning of informal care: Gender and the contribution of elderly people, *Ageing and Society*, 10(4): 429–54.

Arber, S. and Ginn, J. (1991a) *Gender and Later Life: A Sociological Analysis of Resources and Constraints*. London: Sage.

Arber, S. and Ginn, J. (1991b) The invisibility of age: Gender and class in later life, *Sociological Review*, 39(2): 260–91.

Arber, S. and Ginn, J. (1992) Class and caring: A forgotten dimension, *Sociology*, 26(4): 619–34.

Arber, S. and Ginn, J. (1993a) Class, caring and the life-course. In S. Arber and M. Evandrou (eds) *Ageing, Independence and the Life-course*. London: Jessica Kingsley.

Arber, S. and Ginn, J. (1993b) Gender and inequalities in health in later life, *Social Science and Medicine*, 36(1): 33–47.

Arber, S. and Ginn, J. (1995a) The mirage of gender equality: Occupational success in the labour market and within marriage, *British Journal of Sociology*, 46(1): 21–43.

Arber, S. and Ginn, J. (1995b) Gender differences in informal caring, *Health and Social Care in the Community*, 3: 19–31.

Aronson, J. (1990) Women's perspectives on informal care of the elderly: Public ideology and personal experience of giving and receiving care, *Ageing and Society*, 10: 61–84.

Aronson, J. (1992) Women's sense of responsibility for the care of old people: 'But who else is going to do it?' *Gender and Society*, 6: 8–29.

Askham, J. (1984) *Identity and Stability in Marriage*. Cambridge: Cambridge University Press.

Askham, J. (1994) Marriage relationships of older people, *Reviews in Clinical Gerontology*, 4: 261–8.

Askham, J., Henshaw, L. and Tarpey, M. (1993) Policies and perceptions of identity. Service needs of elderly people from black and ethnic minority backgrounds. In S. Arber and M. Evandrou (eds) *Ageing, Independence and the Life Course*. London: Jessica Kingsley Publishers.

Atchley, R. C. (1976) Selected social and psychological differences between men and women in later life, *Journal of Gerontology*, 31: 204–211.

Atchley, R. C. (1982) The process of retirement: Comparing women and men. In M. Szinovacz (ed.) *Women's Retirement*. London: Sage.

Atchley, R. C. (1992) Retirement and marital satisfaction. In M. Szinovacz, D. Ekerdt and B. Vinick (eds) *Families and Retirement*. London: Sage.

Atchley, R. C. (1993) Continuity theory and the evolution of activity in later adulthood. In J. R. Kelly (ed.) *Activity and Aging – Staying Involved in Later Life*. Newbury Park, CA: Sage.

Avison, W. R., Turner, J., Noh, S. and Nixon Speechley, K. (1993) The impact of care-giving: Comparisons of different family contexts and experiences. In S. K. Zarit, L. I. Pearlin and K. Warner Schaie (eds) *Caregiving Systems: Informal and Formal Helpers*. New York: Erlbaum.

Baars, J. (1991) The challenge of critical gerontology: The problem of social constitution, *Journal of Ageing Studies*, 5: 219–43.

Baldwin, S. and Falkingham, J. (eds) (1994) *Social Security and Social Change: New Challenges to the Beveridge Model*. Hemel Hempstead: Harvester Wheatsheaf.

Barrett, M. (1980) *Women's Oppression Today: Problems in Marxist Feminist Analysis*. London: Verso.

Bassein, B. A. (1993) *The Matriarch's Power: A Cross-cultural Literary Study*. New York: Lang.

Bauman, Z. (1992) *Intimations of Postmodernity*. London: Routledge.

Bayley, M., Seyd, R., Tennant, A. and Simons, K. (1982) What resources does the informal sector require to fulfil its role? In *The Barclay Report: Papers from a Consultative Day*. National Institute of Social Work Paper No. 15. London: National Institute of Social Work.

Begum, N. (1991) 'At the mercy of others: Disabled women's experiences of receiving personal care', paper presented at BSA Annual Conference, University of Manchester, Manchester, March.

Bengtson, V. L. (1989) The problem of generations: Age groups, cohorts, continuities and social change. In V. L. Bengtson and K. W. Schaie (eds) *The Course of Later Life*. New York: Springer Publishing Co.

Bennett, G. (1990) Shifting emphasis from abused to abuser, *Geriatric Medicine*, 20(5): 45–47.

Bennett, G. and Kingston, P. (1993) *Elder Abuse: Concepts, Theories and Interventions*. London: Chapman and Hall.

Berger, R. (1982) The unseen minority: Older gays and lesbians, *Social Work*, 27: 236–42.

Bernard, J. (1976) *The Future of Marriage*. Harmondsworth: Penguin.

Bernard, M. and Meade, K. (eds) (1993) *Women Come of Age: Perspectives on the Lives of Older Women*. London: Edward Arnold.

Bhalla, A. and Blakemore, K. (1981) *Elders of the Ethnic Minority Groups*. Birmingham: AFFOR.

Blaikie, A. (1994) Ageing and consumer culture: Will we reap the whirlwind? *Generations Review*, 4(4): 5–7.

Blieszner, R. (1993) A socialist–feminist perspective on widowhood, *Journal of Aging Studies*, 7: 171–82.

Block, M. and Sinnott, J. (1979) Methodology and research. In M. Block and J. Sinnott (eds) *The Battered Elder Syndrome: an exploratory study*. College Park Centre on Ageing, College Park, MD: University of Maryland.

Bone, M., Gregory, J., Gill, B. and Lader, D. (1992) *Retirement and Retirement Plans*. OPCS, London: HMSO.

Borland, K. (1991) 'That's not what I said': Interpretive conflict in oral history narrative research. In S. Gluck and D. Patai (eds) *Women's Words: The Feminist Practice of Oral History*. London: Routledge.

Bott, E. (1957) *Family and Social Network*. London: Tavistock.

Bowling, A., Farquhar, M., Grundy, E. and Formby, J. (1992) 'Psychiatric morbidity among people aged 85+: a follow up study', Working Paper No.1, Age Concern Institute of Gerontology, King's College London.

Briggs, A. and Oliver, J. (eds) (1985) *Caring: The Experience of Looking After Disabled Relatives*. London: Routledge and Kegan Paul.

Briggs, R. (1993) Biological ageing. In J. Bond, P. Coleman and S. Peace (eds) *Ageing in Society*. London: Sage.

Brubaker, T. (1990) Families in later life: A burgeoning research area, *Journal of Marriage and the Family,* 52: 959–81.

Bruce, E. and Rose, H. (1994) 'Secrets and the co-production of social research knowledge of older people's lives', paper presented at Gender and Ageing Symposium, University of Surrey, Guildford, July.

Burgoyne, J. and Clark, D. (1984) *Making a Go of It: A Study of Stepfamilies in Sheffield.* London: Routledge.

Burwell, E. J. (1982) The handwriting is on the wall: Older women in the future, *Resources for Feminist Research,* 11: 208–9.

Burwell, E. J. (1984) Sexism in social science research on aging. In J. M. Vickers (ed.) *Taking Sex into Account.* Ottawa: Carleton University Press.

Bury, M. and Holme, A. (1991) *Life after Ninety.* London: Routledge.

Bury, M., Gabe, J. and Wright, Z. (1994) *Health Promotion and Mental Health.* London: Health Education Authority.

Bytheway, B. (1987) 'Male carers: Questions of intervention', paper presented to conference on Evaluating Support to Informal Carers, Social Policy Research Unit, University of York, York, June.

Bytheway, B. (1995) *Ageism.* Buckingham: Open University Press.

Bytheway, B., Keil, T., Allatt, P. and Bryman, A. (eds) (1989) *Becoming and Being Old: Sociological Approaches to Later Life.* London: Sage.

Calasanti, T. M. (1993) Bringing in diversity: Toward an inclusive theory of retirement, *Journal of Aging Studies,* 7: 133–50.

Calasanti, T. M. and Zajicek, A. M. (1993) A socialist–feminist approach to aging: embracing diversity, *Journal of Aging Studies,* 7: 117–31.

Canadian Study of Health and Aging (1994) Patterns of caring for people with dementia in Canada, *Canadian Journal on Aging,* 13(4): 470–87.

Carby, H. (1982) 'White woman listen': Black feminism and the boundaries of sisterhood. In Centre for Cultural Studies (ed.) *The Empire Strikes Back.* London: Hutchnison.

Carlsen, S. and Larsen, J. (eds) (1993) *The Equality Dilemma. Reconciling Working Life and Family Life, Viewed in an Equality Perspective.* Copenhagen: The Danish Equal Status Council.

Central Statistical Office (1994) *Social Trends 24.* London: HMSO.

Chapman, N. J. (1989) Gender, marital status, and childlessness of older persons and the availability of informal assistance. In M.D. Petersen and D.L. White (eds) *Health Care of the Elderly: An Information Source-book.* Newbury Park : Sage Publications.

Chappell, N. L. and Havens, B. (1980) Old and female: Testing the double jeopardy hypothesis, *The Sociological Quarterly,* 21: 157–71.

Clark, D. (1982) Marriage and remarriage: New wine in old bottles. In S. Saunders (ed.) *Change in Marriage.* Rugby: National Marriage Guidance Council.

Clark, D. (1987) Changing partners: Marriage and divorce across the life course. In G. Cohen (ed.) *Social Change and the Life Course.* London: Tavistock.

Clark, D. (ed.) (1991a) *Marriage, Domestic Life and Social Change: Writings for Jacqueline Burgoyne.* London: Routledge.

Clark, D. (1991b) Constituting the marital world: A qualitative perspective. In D. Clark (ed.) *Marriage, Domestic Life and Social Change.* London: Routledge.

Clark, P. (1993) Public policy in the US and Canada: Individualism, familial obligation and collective responsibility in the care of the elderly. In J. Hendricks and C. J. Rosenthal (eds) *The Remainder of their Days: Domestic Policy and Older Families in the United States and Canada.* New York: Garland Publishing.

Clennell, S. (1987) *Older Students in Adult Education*. Milton Keynes: Open University Press.

Cliff, D. (1993) 'Under the wife's feet': Renegotiating gender divisions in early retirement, *Sociological Review*, 41(1): 30–53.

Clulow, C. (1991) Making, breaking and remaking marriages. In D.Clark (ed.) *Marriage, Domestic Life and Social Change*. London: Routledge.

Cockburn, C. (1991) *In the Way of Women: Men's Resistance to Sex Equality in Organizations*. London: Macmillan.

Coleman, P., Bond, J. and Peace, S. (1993) Ageing in the twentieth century. In J. Bond, P. Coleman and S. Peace (eds) *Ageing in Society*. London: Sage.

Coleman, P. and McCulloch, A. (1985) The study of psychosocial change in late life: Some conceptual and methodological issues. In J. Munnichs, P. Mussen and P. Coleman (eds) *Retirement, Life Span and Change in a Gerontological Perspective*. Orlando, Academic Press.

Connidis, I. A. (1989) *Family Ties and Aging*. Toronto: Butterworths.

Connidis, I. A. and McMullin, J. A. (1993) To have or have not: Parent status and the subjective well-being of older men and women, *The Gerontologist*, 33: 630–6.

Coontz, S. and Henderson, P. (1986) Property forms, political power, and female labour in the origins of class and state societies. In S. Coontz and P. Henderson (eds) *Women's Work, Men's Property*. London: Verso.

Corin, E. (1982) Elderly people's social strategies for survival: A dynamic use of social networks analysis, *Canada's Mental Health*, 30(3): 7–12.

Cornwell, J. (1984) *Hard Earned Lives*. London: Tavistock.

Cowgill, D. O. and Holmes, L. D. (1972) *Aging and Modernization*. New York: Appleton-Century-Crofts.

Crompton, R. and Jones, G. (1984) *White Collar Proletariat*. London: Macmillan.

Crompton, R. and Sanderson, K. (1990) *Gendered Jobs and Social Change*. London: Unwin Hyman.

Cumming, E. and Henry, W. E. (1966) *Growing Old, the Process of Disengagement*. New York: Basic Books.

Cunnison, S. (1987) Women's three working lives and trade union participation. In P. Allatt *et al.* (eds) *Women and the Lifecycle: Transitions and Turning Points*. Basingstoke: Macmillan.

d'Abbs, P. (1982) *Social Support Networks: A Critical Review of Models and Findings*. Melbourne: Institute of Family Studies Monograph No. 1.

Dalley, G. (1988) *Ideologies of Caring: Rethinking Community and Collectivism*. Basingstoke: Macmillan.

Dannefer, D. (1984) Adult development and social theory: A paradigmatic reappraisal, *American Sociological Review*, 49: 100–116.

Davies, B. and Ward, S. (1992) *Women and Personal Pensions*. London: HMSO/Equal Opportunities Commission.

Davies, R., Elias, P. and Penn, R. (1992) The relationship between a husband's unemployment and his wife's participation in the labour force, *Oxford Bulletin of Economics and Statistics*, 54(2): 145–72.

Decalmer, P. and Glendenning, F. (1993) *The Mistreatment of Elderly People*. London: Sage.

Delphy, C. and Leonard, D. (1992) *Familiar Exploitation: A New Analysis of Marriage in Contemporary Western Societies*. Cambridge: Polity Press.

Denton, F. T., Feaver, H. C. and Spencer, B. G. (1987) The Canadian population and labour force: Retrospect and prospect. In V. W. Marshall (ed.) *Aging in Canada: Social Perspectives*. Markham: Fitzhenry and Whiteside.

Department of Employment (1991) *New Earnings Survey, 1991*. London: HMSO.

Department of Health (1989) *Caring for People: Community Care in the Next Decade and Beyond*, White Paper, Cmnd 849. London: HMSO.

Department of Health and Social Security (DHSS) (1981) *Growing Older*, Cmnd 8173. London: HMSO.

Department of Health Social Services Inspectorate (1992) *Confronting Elder Abuse: An SSI London Region Survey*. London: HMSO.

Dobash, R. E. and Dobash, R. P. (1992) *Women, Violence and Social Change*. London: Routledge.

Dressel, P. L. (1991) Gender, race and class: Beyond the feminization of poverty in later life. In M. Minkler and C. L. Estes (eds) *Critical Perspectives on Aging: The Political and Moral Economy of Growing Old*. New York: Baywood.

Drury, E. (1993) *Age Discrimination against Older Workers in the European Community: A Comparative Analysis*. London: Eurolink.

Eastman, M. (1984) *Old Age Abuse*. Mitcham: Age Concern England.

Edwards, M. (1980) Economy of home activities, *Australian Journal of Social Issues*, 15(1): 5–16.

Eekelaar, J. and Pearl, D. (1989) *An Aging World*. Oxford: Clarendon Press.

Elder, G. H. and O'Rand, A. M. (1995). Adult lives in a changing society. In K. Cook, G. Fine and J. S. House (eds) *Sociological Perspectives on Social Psychology*. New York: Allyn Bacon.

Elias, P. and Gregory, M. (1994) *The Changing Structure of Occupations and Earnings in Great Britain, 1975–1990*, Department of Employment, Research Series No 27. Sheffield: Research Strategy Branch.

Eliasson, R. (1989) Perspectives and outlooks in social science research. In A. Elzinga (ed.) *In Science We Trust?* Lund: Lund University Press.

Equal Opportunities Commission (1980) *The Experience of Caring for Elderly and Handicapped Dependants*. Manchester: Equal Opportunities Commission.

Equal Opportunities Commission (1982) *Who Cares for the Carer? Opportunities for Those Caring for the Elderly and Handicapped*. Manchester: Equal Opportunities Commission.

Ermisch, J. (1990) *Fewer Babies, Longer Lives*. York: Joseph Rowntree Foundation.

ESRC Data Archive (1994a) *General Household Surveys 1991 and 1992* [computer files]. Colchester: ESRC Data Archive.

ESRC Data Archive (1994b) *Retirement and Retirement Plans Survey, 1988* [computer files]. Colchester: ESRC Data Archive.

Estes, C. (1986) Politics of ageing in America, *Ageing in Society*, 6(2): 121–34.

Estes, C. (1991) The new political economy of aging: Introduction and critique. In M. Minkler and C. L. Estes (eds) *Critical Perspectives on Aging: The Moral and Political Economy of Growing Old*. New York: Baywood Publishing Co.

Estes, C. L. (1983) Austerity and aging in the United States: 1980 and beyond. In A. Guillemard (ed.) *Old Age and the Welfare State*. Beverly Hills, CA: Sage.

Estes, C. L., Swan, J. H. and Gerard, L. E. (1982) Dominant and competing paradigms in gerontology: Towards a political economy of ageing, *Ageing and Society*, 12: 151–64.

Evandrou, M. and Falkingham, J. (1993) Social security and the life course: Developing sensitive policy alternatives. In S. Arber and M. Evandrou (eds) *Ageing, Independence and the Life Course*. London: Jessica Kingsley Publishers.

Featherstone, M. and Hepworth, M. (1989) Ageing and old age: Reflections on the postmodern life course. In B. Bytheway, T. Keil, P. Allatt and A. Bryman (eds) *Becoming and Being Old: Sociological Approaches to Later Life.* London: Sage.

Featherstone, M. and Hepworth, M. (1991) The mask of ageing and the postmodern life course. In M. Featherstone, M. Hepworth and B. S. Turner (eds) *The Body: Social Process and Cultural Theory.* London: Sage.

Feil, N. (1993) *The Validation Breakthrough.* Baltimore, MD: Health Professions Press.

Fennell, G., Phillipson, C. and Evers, H. (1988) *The Sociology of Old Age.* Milton Keynes: Open University Press.

Filinson, R. and Ingman, S. R. (1989) *Elder Abuse, Practice and Policy.* New York: Human Sciences Press.

Finch, J. (1986) Age. In R. Burgess (ed.) *Key Variables in Social Investigation.* London: Routledge and Kegan Paul.

Finch, J. (1989) *Family Obligations and Social Change.* Cambridge: Polity Press.

Finch, J. and Groves, D. (1980) Community care for the elderly: A case for equal opportunities? *Journal of Social Policy,* 9(4): 487–514.

Finch, J. and Groves, D. (1982) By women for women: Caring for the frail elderly, *Women's Studies International Forum,* 5: 427–38.

Finch, J. and Groves, D. (eds) (1983) *A Labour of Love: Women, Work and Caring.* London: Routledge and Kegan Paul.

Finch, J. and Mason, J. (1993) *Negotiating Family Responsibilities.* London: Routledge.

Finch, J. and Summerfield, P. (1991) Social reconstruction and the emergence of companionate marriage 1945–59. In D. Clark (ed.) *Marriage, Domestic Life and Social Change.* London: Routledge.

Finkelhor, D. and Pillemer, K. (1988) Elder abuse: Its relation to other forms of domestic violence. In G. T. Hotaling, D. Finkelhor, J. T. Kirkpatrick and M. A. Strauss (eds) *Family Abuse and its Consequences: New Directions in Research.* Newbury Park, CA: Sage.

Finley, N. J. (1989) Theories of family labor as applied to gender differences in caregiving for elderly parents, *Journal of Marriage and the Family,* 51: 79–86.

Fisher, M. (1993) 'Man-made care: Community care and older male carers', University of Bristol, mimeo.

Fitting, M., Rabins, P., Lucas, M. and Eastham, J. (1986) Caregivers for dementia patients: A comparison of husbands and wives, *The Gerontologist,* 26(3): 248–52.

Fonow, M. M. and Cook, J. A. (1991) *Beyond Methodology: Feminist Scholarship as Lived Research.* Bloomington, IN: Indiana University Press.

Forster, E. M. (1989) *Howards End.* Harmondsworth: Penguin.

Fox, B. (1988) Conceptualizing 'patriarchy', *Canadian Review of Sociology and Anthropology,* 25: 163–81.

Fox, B. (1989) The feminist challenge: A reconsideration of social inequality and economic development. In R. J. Brym and B. J. Fox (eds) *From Culture to Power: The Sociology of English Canada.* Toronto: Oxford University Press.

Fox, J. A. (1976) 'Women, work and retirement', PhD thesis, Duke University, Durham, NC.

Francis, D. (1984) *Will You Still Need Me, Will You Still Feed Me, When I'm 84?* Bloomington, IN: Indiana University Press.

Friedan, B. (1993) *The Fountain of Age.* New York: Simon and Schuster.

Friedman, A. (1987) Getting powerful with age: Changes in women over the life cycle, *Israel Social Science Research,* 5(1/2): 76–86.

Fry, P. S. (1992) Major social theories of aging and their implications for counselling concepts and practice: A critical review, *The Counselling Psychologist*, 20: 246–329.

Fuchs, W. (1984) *Biographische Forschung. Eine Einführung in die Praxis und Methoden.* Opladen: Westdeutscher Verlag.

Fulmer, T. and O'Malley, T. A. (1987) *Inadequate Care of the Elderly*. New York: Springer.

Gallie, D., Marsh, C. and Vogler, C. (eds) (1994) *The Social Consequences of Unemployment*. Oxford: Oxford University Press.

Gallie, D. and Vogler, C. (1990) Unemployment and attitudes to work, Working Paper No. 18, Oxford: Nuffield College.

Gans, H. (1992) Preface. In M. Lamont and M. Fournier (eds) *Cultivating Differences: Symbolic Boundaries and the Making of Inequality*. Chicago, IL: Chicago University Press.

Gee, E. M. and Kimball, M. M. (1987) *Women and Aging*. Toronto: Butterworths.

Giddens, A. (1991) *Modernity and Self Identity: Self and Society in the Late Modern Age*. Cambridge: Polity Press.

Giddens, A. (1992) *The Transformation of Intimacy*. Cambridge: Polity Press.

Giddens, A. (1994) *Beyond Left and Right: The Future of Radical Politics*. London: Polity Press.

Gilford, R. (1984) Contrasts in marital satisfaction throughout old age: An exchange theory analysis, *Journal of Gerontology*, 39: 325–33.

Gilleard, C. J. (1984) *Living with Dementia: Community Care of the Elderly Mentally Infirm*. London: Croom Helm.

Gilligan, C. (1982) *In a Different Voice: Psychological Theory and Women's Moral Development*. Cambridge, MA: Harvard University Press.

Ginn, J. and Arber, S. (1991) Gender, class and income inequalities in later life, *British Journal of Sociology*, 42(3): 369–96.

Ginn, J. and Arber, S. (1992) Towards women's independence: Pension systems in three contrasting European welfare states, *Journal of European Social Policy*, 4(2): 255–77.

Ginn, J. and Arber, S. (1993) Pension penalties: The gendered division of occupational welfare, *Work, Employment and Society*, 7(1): 47–70.

Ginn, J. and Arber, S. (1994a) Heading for hardship: How the British pension system has failed women. In S. Baldwin and J. Falkingham (eds) *Social Security and Social Change: New Challenges to the Beveridge Model*. Hemel Hempstead: Harvester Wheatsheaf.

Ginn, J. and Arber, S. (1994b) 'Work histories and the occupational pension income of older women and men', paper presented at the Work, Employment and Society Conference, University of Kent, Canterbury, September.

Ginn, J. and Arber, S. (in press) Gender, age and attitudes to retirement, *Ageing and Society*.

Gittins, D. (1985) *The Family in Question: Changing Households and Family Ideologies*. London: Macmillan.

Glendinning, C. (1987) *Impoverishing Women in the Growing Divide*. London: Child Poverty Action Group.

Godkin, M. A., Wolf, R. S. and Pillemer, K. A. (1989) A case-comparison analysis of elder abuse and neglect, *International Journal of Aging and Human Development*, 28(3): 201–25.

Gorey, K. M., Rice, R. W. and Brice, G. C. (1992) The prevalence of elder care responsibilities among the work force population: Response bias among groups of cross-sectional surveys, *Research on Aging*, 14: 399–418.

Gottlieb, B. H., Kelloway, E. K. and Fraboni, M. (1994) Aspects of eldercare that place employees at risk, *The Gerontologist*, 34(6): 815–27.

Gove, W. R. and Tudor, J. F. (1973) Adult sex roles and mental illness. *American Journal of Sociology*, 78(4): 810–21.

Green, H. (1988) *Informal Carers*, OPCS Series GHS, No.15, Supplement A, London: HMSO.

Green, H. (1990) Survey of carers: Methodological problems, *Survey Methodology Bulletin*, 26: 17–25. OPCS. London: HMSO.

Greene, V. (1989) Human capitalism and intergenerational justice, *The Gerontologist*, 29(6): 723–4.

Groves, D. and Finch, J. (1983) Natural selection: Perspectives on entitlement to the invalid care allowance. In D. Groves and J. Finch (eds) *A Labour of Love: Women, Work and Caring*. London: Routledge and Kegan Paul.

Gubrium, J. F. (1986) *Oldtimers and Alzheimer's: The Descriptive Organisation of Senility*. London: JAI Press.

Guillemard, A. (ed.) (1983) *Old Age and the Welfare State*. Beverly Hills, CA: Sage.

Gunaratnam, Y. (1993) Breaking the silence: Asian carers in Britain. In J. Bornat, C. Pereira, D. Pilgrim and F. Williams (eds) *Community Care: A Reader*. Basingstoke: Macmillan.

Gutmann, D. (1987) *Reclaimed Powers: Toward a New Psychology of Men and Women in Later Life*. New York: Basic Books.

Handy, C. (1991) *The Age of Unreason*. London: Century Business.

Hanmer, J. (1990) Men, power and the exploitation of women. In J. Hearn and D. Morgan (eds) *Men, Masculinities and Social Theory*. London: Unwin.

Hanmer, J. and Hearn, J. (1994) 'Theory and research on violence', paper presented at Violence, Gender and Social Work Conference, University of Bradford, Bradford, March.

Hareven, T. K. and Adams, K. J. (1982) *Ageing and Life Course Transitions*. London: Tavistock.

Harrop, A. (1990) *The Employment Position of Older Women in Europe*. London: Age Concern/Institute of Gerontology, King's College.

Hartmann, H. (1981) The unhappy marriage of Marxism and feminism: Towards a more progressive union. In L. Sargent (ed.) *Women and Revolution*. Boston, MA: South End Press.

Hartsock, N. (1983) *Money, Sex, and Power: Toward A Feminist Historical Materialism*. Boston, MA: Northeastern University Press.

Havinghurst, R. J. (1954) Flexibility and the social roles of the retired, *American Journal of Sociology*, 59: 309–11.

Hearn, J., Sheppard, D., Tancred-Sheriff, P. and Burrell, G. (1989) *The Sexuality of Organization*. London: Sage.

Hen Co-op (1993) *Growing Old Disgracefully*. London: Piatkus.

Henderson, J. (1988) 'Conceptualisation of informal care: An analysis of community care policies based on the perceptions of informal carers of elderly women', unpublished PhD Thesis. University of Bradford, Bradford.

Hendricks, J. (1993) Recognizing the relativity of gender in aging research, *Journal of Aging Studies*, 7: 111–16.

Hendricks, J. and Rosenthal, C. J. (eds) (1993) *The Remainder of their Days: Domestic Policy and Older Families in the United States and Canada*. New York: Garland Publishing.

Henretta, J. (1994) Recent trends in retirement, *Reviews in Clinical Gerontology*, 4: 71–81.

Henretta, J. and O'Rand, A. (1983) Joint retirement in the dual worker family, *Social Forces*, 62(2): 504–20.

Henwood, M., Rimmer, L. and Wicks, M. (1987) *Inside the Family: Changing Roles of Men and Women*, occasional paper. London: Family Policy Studies Centre.

Herz, D. and Rones, P. (1989) Institutional barriers to employment of older women, *Monthly Labor Review*, 112(4): 14–21.

Hess, B. B. (1985) Aging policies and old women: The hidden agenda. In A. S. Rossi (ed.) *Gender and the Life Course*. New York: Aldine.

Hess, B. B. (1986) Antidiscrimination policies today and the life chances of older women tomorrow, *Gerontologist*, 26(2): 132–5.

Hess, B. B. (1990) Gender and aging: The demographic parameters, *Generations*, 14: 12–15.

Hicks, C. (1988) *Who Cares? Looking After People at Home*. London: Virago.

Hirschorn, L. (1977) Postindustrial life: A US perspective, *Futures*, 287–98.

HMSO (1994) *Equality in State Pension Age*, Cm 2420. London: HMSO.

Hochschild, A. (1983) *The Managed Heart: The Commercialization of Human Feelings*. Berkeley, CA: University of California Press.

Hochschild, A. (1990) *The Second Shift: Working Parents and the Revolution at Home*. London: Piatkus.

Hockey, J. and James, A. (1993) *Growing Up and Growing Old: Ageing, Dependency and the Life Course*. London: Sage.

Holt, M. (1993) Elder sexual abuse in Britain: Preliminary findings, *Journal of Elder Abuse and Neglect*, 5(2): 63–71.

Homer, A. and Gilleard, C. (1990) Abuse of elderly people by their carers, *British Medical Journal*, 301: 1359–62.

Hudson, M. F. (1986) Elder mistreatment: Current research. In K. A. Pillemer and R. Wolf (eds) *Elder Abuse: Conflict in the Family*. Dover, MA: Auburn House.

Hunt, A. (1978) *The Elderly at Home*. OPCS, London: HMSO.

Itzin, C. (1986) Media images of women: The social construction of ageism and sexism. In S. Wilkinson (ed.) *Feminist Social Psychology*. Milton Keynes: Open University Press.

Itzin, C. (1990a) 'Age and sexual divisions: A study of opportunity and identity in women', PhD thesis, University of Kent.

Itzin, C. (1990b) As old as you feel. In P. Thompson, C. Itzin and M. Abendstern (eds) *I Don't Feel Old: The Experience of Later Life*. Oxford: Oxford University Press.

Itzin, C. and Newman, J. (1995) *Gender, Culture and Organizational Change: Putting Theory into Practice*. London: Routledge.

Itzin, C. and Phillipson, C. (1993) *Age Barriers at Work: Maximising the Potential of Mature and Older People*. Solihull: Metropolitan Authorities Recruitment Agency (METRA).

Itzin, C. and Phillipson, C. (1995) The double jeopardy of age and gender. In C. Itzin and J. Newman (eds) *Gender, Culture and Organizational Change: Putting Theory into Practice*. London: Routledge.

Jacobson, D. (1974) Rejection of the retiree role: A study of female industrial workers in their 50s, *Human Relations*, 27: 477–491.

Jaggar, A. (1983) *Feminist Politics and Human Nature*. Ottawa: Rowman and Allanheld.

James, N. (1989) Emotional labour: Skill and work in the regulation of feelings, *Sociological Review*, 37(1): 15–42.

James, N. (1992) Care = organization + physical labour + emotional labour, *Sociology of Health and Illness*, 14: 488–509.

Jefferys, M. (ed.) (1989) *Growing Old in the Twentieth Century*. London: Routledge.

Jerrome, D. (1989) Virtue and vicissitude: The role of old people's clubs. In M. Jefferys (ed.) *Growing Old in the Twentieth Century*. London: Routledge.

Jerrome, D. (1990) Intimate relationships. In J. Bond and P. Coleman (eds) *Ageing in Society: An Introduction to Social Gerontology*. London: Sage.

Jerrome, D. (1993) *Good Company*. Edinburgh: Edinburgh University Press.

Johnson, C. (1985) The impact of illness on later life marriages, *Journal of Marriage and the Family*, 47: 165–72.

Johnson, C. L. and Barer, B. M. (1992) Patterns of engagement and disengagement among the oldest old, *Journal of Aging Studies*, 6(4): 351–64.

Johnson, P., Conrad, C. and Thomson, D. (1989) *Workers versus Pensioners: Intergenerational Justice in an Ageing World*. Manchester: Manchester University Press.

Jones, K. (1990) Citizenship in a woman friendly polity, *Signs: Journal of Women in Culture and Society*, 15(4): 781–812.

Jowell, R., Witherspoon, S. and Brook, L. (eds) (1990) *British Social Attitudes: 7th Report*. Aldershot: SCPR/Gower.

Kaden, J. and McDaniel, S. A. (1990) Caregiving and care-receiving: A double bind for women in Canada's aging society, *Journal of Women and Aging*, 2(3): 3–26.

Katz, S., Ford, A. B., Moskowitz, R. W., Jackson, B. A. and Jaffe, M. W. (1963) Studies of illness in the aged: The index of ADL, a standardized measure of biological and psychosocial function, *Journal of the American Medical Association*, 185: 914–19.

Keith, P. and Schafer, R. (1982) Employment status, household involvement and psychological well-being of men and women, *International Journal of Sociology of the Family*, 12(1): 101–10.

Keith, P. and Wacker, R. (1990) Sex roles in the older family. In T. Brubaker (ed.) *Family Relationships in Later Life*, 2nd edn. London: Sage.

Keith, P. M. (1989) *The Unmarried in Later Life*. New York: Praeger.

Kelly, L. (1988) *Surviving Sexual Violence*. Cambridge: Polity Press.

Kelly, L., Burton, S. and Regan, L. (1994) Researching women's lives or studying women's oppression? Reflections on what constitutes feminist research. In M. Maynard and J. Purvis (eds) *Researching Women's Lives from a Feminist Perspective*. London: Taylor and Francis.

Kendig, H. (1986) Family and network structure. In H. Kendig (ed.) *Ageing and Families: A Support Networks Perspective*. Boston, MA: Allen and Unwin.

Kohli, M. (1988) Ageing as a challenge for sociological theory, *Ageing and Society*, 8(4): 367–94.

Kohli, M. and Meyer, J. W. (1986) Social structure and the social construction of life stages, *Human Development*, 29: 145–80.

Kohli, M. and Rein, M. (1991) The changing balance of work and retirement. In M. Kohli, M. Rein, A-M. Guillemard and H. Gunsteren (eds) *Time for Retirement: Comparative Studies of Early Exit from the Labor Force*. Cambridge: Cambridge University Press.

Kohli, M., Rein, M., Guillemard, A-M. and Gunsteren, H. (eds) (1991) *Time for Retirement: Comparative Studies of Early Exit from the Labor Force*. Cambridge: Cambridge University Press.

Kohli, M., Rosenow, J. and Wolf, J. (1983) The social construction of ageing through work: Economic structure and life-world, *Ageing and Society*, 3: 23–42.

Kyle, I. (1993) 'Private and public discourses: Socio-historical contexts of child care', unpublished manuscript. Department of Family Studies, University of Guelph, Guelph, Ontario, Canada.

Laczko, F. (1990) New poverty and the old poor: Pensioners' incomes in the European Community, *Ageing and Society*, 10(3): 261–78.

Laczko, F. and Phillipson, C. (1991) *Changing Work and Retirement: Social Policy and the Older Worker*. Milton Keynes: Open University Press.

Land, H. and Rose, H. (1985) Compulsory altruism or an altruistic society for all? In P. Bean, J. Ferris and D. Whynes (eds) *In Defence of Welfare*. London: Tavistock.

Laslett, P. (1987) The emergence of the third age, *Ageing and Society*, 7(2): 133–60.

Laslett, P. (1989a) *A Fresh Map of Life: The Emergence of the Third Age*. London: Weidenfeld & Nicolson.

Laslett, P. (1989b) The demographic scene – an overview. In J. Eekelaar and D. Pearl (eds) *An Ageing World: Dilemmas and Challenges for Law and Social Policy*. Oxford: Clarendon Press.

Lawson, A. (1988) *Adultery: An Analysis of Love and Betrayal*. New York: Basic Books.

Lee, G. (1988) Marital satisfaction in later life: The effects of non-marital roles, *Journal of Marriage and the Family*, 50: 775–83.

Lee, G. and Shehan, C. (1989) Retirement and marital satisfaction, *Journal of Gerontology*, 44: S226–30.

Lemmer, E. M. (1991) Untidy careers: Occupational profiles of re-entry women, *International Journal of Career Management*, 3(1): 13–17.

Leonard, F. (1982) Not even for dogcatcher: Employment discrimination and older women, *Gray Paper No 8*, Washington DC: Older Women's League.

Levy, J. (1988) Intersections of gender and ageing, *Sociological Quarterly*, 29(4): 479–86.

Lewis, J. and Meredith, B. (1988) *Daughters Who Care: Daughters Caring For Mothers at Home*. London: Routledge.

Lilley, P. (1992) Speech to the International Conference on Social Security Fifty Years after Beveridge, 27 September, York, published as a press release.

Lipp, C. (1988) Überlegungen zur Methodendiskussion. Kulturanthropologische, sozialwissenschaftliche und historische Ansätze zur Erforschung der Geschlechterbeziehungen. In Arbeitsgruppe volkskundliche Frauenforschung Freiburg (eds) *Frauenalltag – Frauenforschung*. Frankfurt: Lang.

Lowenthal, M. and Robinson, B. (1976) Social networks and isolation. In R. Binstock and E. Shanas (eds) *Handbook of Aging and the Social Sciences*. New York: van Nostrand Rheinhold.

Lupri, E. and Frideres, J. (1981) The quality of marriage and the passage of time: Marital satisfaction over the family life cycle, *Canadian Journal of Sociology*, 6: 283–305.

McAllister, L. and Fischer, C. S. (1978) A procedure for surveying personal networks, *Sociological Methods and Research*, 7(2): 131–48.

MacBride-King, J. L. (1990) 'Work and family: Employment challenge of the 90s', Report No. 59–90. Ottawa: The Conference Board of Canada, The Compensation Research Centre.

McConnell, S. (1983) Age discrimination in employment. In H. Parnes (ed.) *Policy Issues in Work and Retirement*. Kalamazoo, MI: W. E. Upjohn Institute for Employment Research.

McCreadie, C. (1991) *Elder Abuse: An Exploratory Study*. London: Age Concern Institute of Gerontology.

McDaniel, S. (1986) *Canada's Aging Population*. Toronto: Butterworths.

McDaniel, S. (1988) *Getting Older and Better: Women and Gender Assumptions in Canada's Aging Society*. Feminist Perspectives, paper no. 11, Ontario: Canadian Research Institute for the Advancement of Women.

McDaniel, S. (1989) Women and ageing: A Sociological perspective, *Journal of Women and Ageing*, 1: 47–67.

MacDonald, B. and Rich, C. (1984) *Look Me in the Eye: Old women, Ageing and Ageism.* San Francisco, CA: Spinsters Ink and London: Women's Press.

McGlone, F. and Cronin, N. (1994) *A Crisis in Care? The Future of Family and State Care for Older People in the European Union.* London: Family Policy Studies Centre.

McKee, L. (1987) Households during unemployment: The resourcefulness of the unemployed. In J. Brannen and G. Wilson (eds) *Give and Take in Families: Studies in Resource Distribution.* London: Allen and Unwin.

McKee, L. and Bell, C. (1985) Marital and family relations in times of male unemployment. In B. Roberts, R. Finnegan and D. Gallie (eds) *New Approaches to Economic Life.* Manchester: Manchester University Press.

McKee, P.L. (1982) *Philosophical Foundations of Gerontology.* New York: Human Sciences Press.

McMullin, J. A. and Ballantyne, P. (1994) 'Employment characteristics and income: Assessing gender and age group effects for Canadians aged 45 years and older', paper presented at the Canadian Sociology and Anthropology Association 29th Annual Meeting, Calgary, June.

Macnicol, J. (1990) Old age and structured dependency. In M. Bury and J. Macnicol (eds) *Aspects of Ageing: Essays on Social Policy and Old Age.* Egham, Royal Holloway University of London: Department of Social Policy and Social Science.

MacPherson, B. (1990) *Aging as a Social Process,* Toronto: Butterworths.

MacRae, H. (1994) 'Managing feeling: Caregiving as emotion work', paper presented to the Annual Meetings of the Canadian Association on Gerontology, Winnipeg, Manitoba, October.

McRobbie, A. (1982) The politics of feminist research: Between talk, text and action, *Feminist Review,* 12: 46–57.

Mannheim, K. (1952) The problem of generations. In K. Mannheim, *Essays on the Sociology of Knowledge,* ed. P. Kecskemeti. London: Routledge and Kegan Paul.

Mansfield, P. and Collard, J. (1988) *The Beginning of the Rest of Your Life: A Portrait of Newly-wed Marriage.* London: Macmillan.

Marsden, D. and Abrams, S. (1987) 'Liberators', 'companions', 'intruders' and 'cuckoos in the nest': A sociology of caring relationships over the life cycle. In P. Allatt, T. Keil, A. Bryman and B. Bytheway (eds) *Women and the Life Cycle: Transitions and Turning Points.* London: Macmillan.

Marshall, V. W. (1987a) Introduction: Social perspectives on aging, in V. W. Marshall (ed.) *Aging in Canada: Social Perspectives.* Markham: Fitzhenry and Whiteside.

Marshall, V. W. (1987b) *Aging in Canada: Social Perspectives.* Markham: Fitzhenry and Whiteside.

Marshall, V. W. (1987c) Social perspective on aging: Theoretical notes. In V. W. Marshall (ed.) *Aging in Canada: Social Perspectives.* Markham: Fitzhenry and Whiteside.

Martin, B. (1990) The cultural construction of ageing: Or how long can the summer wine really last? In M. Bury and J. Macnicol (eds) *Aspects of Ageing: Essays on Social Policy and Old Age.* Egham, Royal Holloway University of London: Department of Social Policy and Social Science.

Martin, J. and Roberts, C. (1984) *Women and Employment: A Lifetime Perspective.* London: HMSO.

Martin Matthews, A. (1993) Issues in the examination of the care giving relationship. In S. H. Zarit, L. I. Pearlin and K. W. Schaie (eds) *Caregiving Systems: Informal and Formal Helpers.* Hillsdale, NJ: Lawrence Erlbaum Associates.

Martin Matthews, A. and Rosenthal, C. J. (1993) Balancing work and family in an aging society: The Canadian experience. In G. L. Maddox and M. P. Lawton (eds) *Annual Review of Gerontology and Geriatrics: Focus on Kinship, Aging and Social Change.* New York: Springer Publishing Company.

Martin Matthews, A. and Rosenthal, C. J. (1994) Women, work and caregiving: How much difference does a great job really make? paper presented at the Annual Scientific and Educational Meetings of the Canadian Association on Gerontology, Winnipeg, October.

Mason, J. (1987) A bed of roses? Women, marriage and inequality in later life. In P. Allatt, T. Keil, A. Bryman and B. Bytheway (eds) *Women and the Life Cycle: Transitions and Turning Points.* London: Macmillan.

Matthews, S. H. (1986) *Friendship through the Life Course.* Beverly Hills, CA: Sage.

Matthews, S. H. and Rosner, T. T. (1988) Shared filial responsibility: The family as the primary caregiver, *Journal of Marriage and the Family,* 50: 185–95.

Mellor, P. (1993) Death in high modernity: The contemporary presence and absence of death. In D. Clark (ed) *The Sociology of Death.* Oxford: Blackwell.

Mills, A. J. (1989) Gender, sexuality and organization theory. In J. Hearn, D. Sheppard, P. Tancred-Sheriff and G. Burrell (eds) *The Sexuality of Organization.* London: Sage.

Milner, J. (1993) A disappearing act: The differing career paths of fathers and mothers in child protection investigations. *Critical Social Policy,* 13(2): 48–68.

Minkler, M. and Cole, T. C. (1991) Political and moral economy: Not such strange bedfellows. In M. Minkler and C. Estes (eds) *Critical Perspectives on Aging.* Amityville, NY: Baywood Publishing Company.

Minkler, M. and Estes, C. (eds) (1991) *Critical Perspectives on Aging.* Amityville, NY: Baywood Publishing Company.

Mirza, K. (1991) Community care for the black community – Waiting for guidance. In Central Council for Education and Training in Social Work (ed.) *One Small Step Towards Racial Justice: the Teaching of Anti-Racism in Social Work Diploma Programmes,* paper 8. London: CCETSW.

Mitterauer, M. and Sieder, R. (1982) *The European Family.* Oxford: Basil Blackwell.

Montgomery, R. J. V. and McGlinn, M. (1992) Women and men in the caregiving role. In L. Glasse and J. Hendricks (eds) *Gender and Aging.* Amityville, NY: Baywood Publishing Company.

Moody, H. R. (1988) Toward a critical gerontology: The contribution of the humanities to theories of aging. In J. E. Birren and V. L. Bengtson (eds) *Emergent Theories of Aging.* New York: Springer Publishing Company.

Morgan, D. (1985) *The Family, Politics and Social Theory.* London: Routledge.

Morgan, D. (1986) Gender. In R. Burgess (ed.) *Key Variables in Social Investigation.* London: Routledge and Kegan Paul.

Morgan, D. (1991) Ideologies of marriage and family life. In D. Clark (ed) *Marriage, Domestic Life and Social Change.* London: Routledge.

Morgan, G. (1986) *Images of Organization.* London: Sage Books.

Morris, L. (1989) Household strategies: The individual, the collective and the labour market – the case of married couples, *Work, Employment and Society,* 3: 447–64.

Morris, L. (1990) *The Workings of the Household.* Cambridge: Polity Press.

Mouser, N., Powers, E., Keith, P. and Goudy, W. (1985) Marital status and life satisfaction: A study of older men. In W. Peterson and J. Quadagno (eds) *Social Bonds in Later Life.* Beverly Hills, CA: Sage.

Mouzelis, N. P. (1991) *Back to Sociological Theory*. London: Macmillan.

Mugford, S. and Kendig, H. (1986) Social relations: Networks and ties. In H. Kendig (ed.) *Ageing and Families: A Support Networks Perspective*. Boston, MA: Allen and Unwin.

Mulqueen, M. (1992) *On Our Own Terms: Redefining Competence and Feminity*. Albany, NY: State University of New York Press.

Myerhoff, B. (1978) *Number Our Days*. New York: Simon and Schuster.

Myles, J. (1989) *Old Age in the Welfare State: The Political Economy of Public Pensions*. Lawrence, KS: The University Press of Kansas.

Nelson, M. (1994) Family day care providers: Dilemmas of daily practice. In E. N. Glenn, G. Chang and L. R. Forcey (eds) *Mothering: Ideology, Experience and Agency*. London: Routledge.

Nelson, S. (1987) *Incest: Fact and Myth*. Edinburgh: Stramullion.

Nett, E. (1982) A call for feminist correctives to research on elders, *Resources for Feminist Research*, 11: 225–6.

Nicholson, J. (1980) *Seven Ages*. London: Fontana.

Nissel, M. and Bonnerjea, L. (1982) *Family Care of the Elderly: Who Pays?* London: Policy Studies Institute.

Noddings, N. (1984) *Caring; A Feminine Approach to Ethics and Moral Education*. Berkeley, CA: University of California Press.

Noe, R.A. (1988) Women and mentoring: A review and research agenda, *Academy of Management Journal*, 18(1): 65–78.

Oakley, A. (1974) *The Sociology of Housework*. London: Pitman Press.

Oakley, A. (1981) Interviewing women: A contradiction in terms. In H. Roberts (ed.) *Doing Feminist Research*. London: Routledge and Kegan Paul.

Oakley, A. (1982) *Subject Women*. London: Fontana.

Oakley, A. (1987) Gender and generation: The life and times of Adam and Eve. In P. Allatt, T. Keil, A. Bryman and B. Bytheway (eds) *Women and the Life Cycle: Transitions and Turning Points*. London: Macmillan.

Ogg, J. (1993) Researching elder abuse, *Ageing and Society*, 13: 389–413.

OPCS (1992) *General Household Survey 1990*. London: HMSO.

OPCS (1988–92) *General Household Survey, 1988–92*, Data files, ESRC Data Archive, University of Essex, Colchester.

Opie, A. (1992) Qualitative research, appropriation of the 'other' and empowerment, *Feminist Review*, 40: 52–69.

O'Rand, A., Henretta, J. and Krecker, M (1992) Family pathways to retirement. In M. Szinovacz, D. Ekerdt and B. Vinick (eds) *Families and Retirement*. Newbury Park, CA: Sage.

Pahl, J. (1989) *Money and Marriage*. Basingstoke: Macmillan Education.

Pahl, J. (1990) Household spending, personal spending and the control of money in marriage, *Sociology*, 24(1): 119–38.

Palo Stoller, E. (1993) Gender and the organization of lay health care: A socialist-feminist perspective, *Journal of Aging Studies*, 7: 151–70.

Parker, R. (1981) Tending and social policy. In E. Goldberg and S. Hatch (eds) *A New Look at the Social Services*. Discussion Paper No. 4. London: Policy Studies Institute.

Parton, N. (1985) *The Politics of Child Abuse*. London: Macmillan.

Peace, S. (1986) The forgotten female: Social policy and older women. In C. Phillipson and A. Walker (eds) *Ageing and Social Policy: A Critical Assessment*. Aldershot: Gower.

Phillips, L. R. (1986) Theoretical explanations of elder abuse. In K. A. Pillemer and R. S Wolf (eds) *Elder Abuse: Conflict in the Family*. Dover, MA: Auburn House.

Phillipson, C. (1993a) Abuse of older people: Sociological perspectives. In P. Decalmer and F. Glendenning (eds) *The Mistreatment of Elderly People*. London: Sage.

Phillipson, C. (1993b) Approaches to advocacy. In M. Bernard and F. Glendenning (eds) *Advocacy, Consumerism and the Older Person*. Stoke-on-Trent: Beth Johnson Foundation.

Phillipson, C. (1994) The modernization of the life course: Implications for social security and older people. In S. Baldwin and J. Falkingham (eds) *Social Security and Social Change*. Hemel Hempstead: Harvester Wheatsheaf.

Pillemer, K. (1986) Risk factors in elder abuse. In K. A. Pillemer and R. S. Wolf (eds) *Elder Abuse: Conflict in the Family*. Dover, MA: Auburn House.

Pillemer, K. A. and Finkelhor, D. (1988) Elder abuse, *The Gerontologist*, 28: 51–57.

Pillemer, K. A. and Finkelhor, D.(1989) Causes of elder abuse: Caregiver stress versus problem relatives, *American Journal of Orthopsychiatry*, 59(2): 179–87.

Pillemer, K. A. and Suitor, J. (1988) Elder abuse. In V. Van Hasselt, R. Morrison, V. Belack and M. Hensen (eds) *Handbook of Family Violence*. New York: Plenum Press.

Pillemer, K. A. and Wolf, R. (eds). (1986) *Elder Abuse: Conflict in the Family*. Dover, MA: Auburn House.

Posner, J. (1977) Old and female: The double whammy, *Essence*, 2: 41–8.

Pritchard, J. (1992) *The Abuse of Elderly People: A Handbook for Professionals*. London: Jessica Kingsley.

Quadagno, J. (1988) Women's access to pensions and the structure of eligibility rules: Systems of production and reproduction, *The Sociological Quarterly*, 29: 541–58.

Quinn, M. J. and Tomita, S. K. (1986) *Elder Abuse and Neglect: Causes, Diagnosis and Intervention Strategies*. New York: Springer.

Quinn, W. H., Hughston, G. A. and Hunter, D. J. (1984) Preservation of independence through non-formal support systems: Implications and promise. In W. H. Quinn and G. A. Hughston (eds) *Independent Aging: Family and Social Systems Perspectives*. Tunbridge Wells: Aspen Systems Corporation.

Quirouette, C. and Gold, D. (1992) Spousal characteristics as predictors of well-being in older couples, *International Journal of Aging and Human Development*, 34: 257–69.

Qureshi, H. and Walker, A. (1989) *The Caring Relationship: Elderly People and Their Families*. Basingstoke: Macmillan.

Rawlins, W. K. (1992) *Friendship Matters: Communication, Dialectics and the Life Course*. New York: Aldine de Gruyter.

Reedy, M., Birren, J. and Schaie, K. (1981) Age and sex differences in satisfying love relationships across the adult life span, *Human Development*, 24: 52–66.

Reinharz, S. (1983) Experiential analysis: A contribution to feminist research. In G. Bowles and R. Klein (eds) *Theories of Women's Studies*. London: Routledge and Kegan Paul.

Reinharz, S. (1986) Friends or foes: Gerontological and feminist theory, *Women's Studies International Forum*, 9: 503–14.

Reinharz, S. (1989) Feminism and anti-ageism: Emergent connections. In A. Herzog, K. Holden and M. Seltzer (eds) *Health and Economic Status of Older Women*. New York: Baywood.

Reskin, B. and Padavic, I. (1994) *Women and Men at Work*. Thousand Oaks, CA: Pine Forge Press.

Rexroat, C. and Shehan, C. (1987) The family life cycle and spouses' time in housework, *Journal of Marriage and the Family*, 49: 737–50.

Ribbens, J. (1989) Interviewing: An unnatural situation, *Women's Studies International Forum*, 12: 579–92.

Richards, T., Richards, L., McGalliard, J. and Sharrock, B. (1992) *Nudist.* Bundorra, Australia: La Trobe University.

Riley, M. W. (1985) Women, men and the lengthening life course. In A. S. Rossi (ed.) *Gender and the Life Course.* New York: Aldine Publishing Co.

Riley, M. W. (1987) On the significance of age in sociology, *American Sociological Review,* 52: 1–14.

Riley, M. W., Foner, A. and Waring, J (1988) Sociology of age. In N. J. Smelser (ed.) *Handbook of Sociology.* London: Sage.

Riley, P. (1983) A structuralist account of political culture, *Administrative Science Quarterly,* 28: 414–37.

Roberts, H. (ed.) (1981) *Doing Feminist Research.* London: Routledge and Kegan Paul.

Rodeheaver, D. (1990) Labor market progeria: On the life expectancy of presentability among working women. In L. Glasse and J. Hendricks (eds) *Gender and Aging.* New York: Baywood.

Rose, H. (1983) Hand, brain and heart, *Signs: Journal of Women in Culture and Society,* 9(3): 73–96.

Rose, H. (1994) *Love, Power and Knowledge: Towards A Feminist Transformation of the Sciences.* Polity Press: Cambridge.

Rosenmayr, L. (1982) Biography and identity. In T. K. Hareven and K. J. Adams (eds) *Ageing and Life Course Transitions: an Interdisciplinary Perspective.* London: Tavistock.

Rosser, C. and Harris, C. (1965) *The Family and Social Change.* London: Routledge and Kegan Paul.

Rossi, A. (1980) Life span theories and women's lives, *Signs,* 6(1): 4–32.

Rossi, A. (1986) Sex and gender in an aging society, *Daedalus,* 115: 141–69.

Ruddick, S. (1982) Maternal thinking. In B. Thorne and M. Yalom (eds) *Rethinking the Family.* London: Longman.

Ruddick, S. (1989) *Maternal Thinking: Towards a Politics of Peace.* Boston, MA: Beacon.

Schuller, T. (1989) Work-ending: Employment and ambiguity in later life. In B. Bytheway, T. Keil, P. Allatt and A. Bryman (eds) *Becoming and Being Old.* London: Sage.

Scott, A. and Wenger, G. C. (1994) *The Impact of Dementia on Support Networks,* research report. Bangor: Centre for Social Policy Research and Development, University of Wales.

Scrutton, S. (1992) *Ageing, Healthy and in Control.* London: Chapman and Hall.

Sengstock, M. C. and Liang, J. (1982) 'Identifying and characterizing elder abuse', unpublished manuscript. Wayne State University, Detroit, MI.

Sharpe, S. (1984) *Double Identity.* Harmondsworth: Penguin.

Shaw, L. (1984) Retirement plans of middle-aged married women, *The Gerontologist,* 24(2): 154–9.

Simonen, L. (1990) Caring by the welfare state and the women behind it: Contradictions and theoretical considerations. In L. Simonen (ed.) *Finnish Debates on Women's Studies.* Tampere: University of Tampere.

Simpson, S. *et al.* (1987) Relationship of supervisors' sex-role stereotypes to performance evaluation of male and female subordinates in non-traditional jobs, *Canadian Journal of Administrative Sciences,* 4(1): 15–30.

Sinnott, J. (1977) Sex-role inconstancy, biology and successful aging, *The Gerontologist,* 17: 459–63.

Sinnott, J. (1986) *Sex Roles and Aging: Theory and Research from a Systems Perspective.* Basle: Karger.

Skucha, J., Bernard, M. and Phillipson, C. (in press) *Women and Work: Implications for Pre-Retirement Education.* Guildford Pre-Retirement Association of Great Britain and Northern Ireland.

Smith, L. J. F. (1989) *Domestic Violence: An Overview of the Literature,* Home Office Research Unit. London: HMSO.

Social Security Advisory Committee (1992) *Options for Equality in State Pension Age: A Case for Equalising at 65.* London: HMSO.

Sontag, S. (1978) The double standard of aging. In V. Carver and P. Liddiard (eds) *An Ageing Population.* London: Hodder and Stoughton.

Stacey, M. (1989) Older women and feminism: A note about my experience of the WLM, *Feminist Review,* 31: 140–2.

Stanley, L. and Wise, S. (1983) *Breaking Out: Feminist Consciousness and Feminist Research.* London, Routledge and Kegan Paul.

Stanley, L. and Wise, S. (1990) *Feminist Praxis: Research, Theory and Epistemology in Feminist Sociology.* London: Routledge.

Stearns, P. (1977) *Old Age in European Society.* London: Croom Helm.

Stearns, P. (1986) Old age family conflict: The perspective of the past. In K. A. Pillemer and R. S. Wolf (eds) *Elder Abuse: Conflict in the Family.* Dover, MA: Auburn House.

Stevenson, O. (1989) *Age and Vulnerability: A Guide to Better Care.* London: Edward Arnold.

Stone, R. (1989) The feminization of poverty among the elderly, *Women's Studies Quarterly,* 1, 2: 20–34.

Stone, R. (1991) Defining family caregivers of the elderly: Implications for research and public policy, *The Gerontologist,* 31: 724–5.

Stone, R., Cafferata, G. L. and Sangl, J. (1987) Caregivers of the frail elderly: A national profile, *The Gerontologist,* 27: 616–26.

Stone, R. and Kemper, P. (1989) Spouses and children of disabled elders: How large a constituency for long-term carereform? *The Milbank Quarterly,* 67: 485–506.

Stone, R. and Minkler, M. (1984) The socio-political context of women's retirement. In M. Minkler and C. Estes (eds) *Political Economy of Aging.* New York: Baywood Publishing Co.

Stott, M. (1981) *Ageing for Beginners.* Oxford: Blackwell.

Streib, G. and Schneider, C. J. (1971) *Retirement in American Society.* Ithaca, NY: Cornell University Press.

Suzman, R. M., Willis, D. P. and Manton, K. G. (eds) (1992) *The Oldest Old.* New York and Oxford: Oxford University Press.

Szinovacz, M. (ed.) (1982) *Women's Retirement: Policy Implications of Recent Research.* Beverly Hills, CA: Sage.

Szinovacz, M. (1987) Preferred retirement timing and retirement satisfaction in women, *International Journal of Aging and Human Development,* 24(4): 301–17.

Szinovacz, M. (1989) Decision-making on retirement timing. In D. Brinberg and J. Jaccard (eds) *Dyadic Decision Making.* New York: Springer-Verlag.

Szinovacz, M. (1991) Women and retirement. In B. Hess and E. Markson (eds) *Growing Old in America.* New York: Transaction Publishers.

Szinovacz, M., Ekerdt, D. and Vinick, B. (eds) (1992) *Families and Retirement.* Newbury Park, CA: Sage.

Taraborrelli, P. (1993) Becoming a carer. In N. Gilbert (ed.) *Researching Social Life*. London: Sage.

Taueber, C. and Valdisera, V. (1986) Women in the American economy. *Current Population Reports*, series p-23, no. 146, Government Printing Office. Washington DC: US Bureau of the Census.

Taylor, R. and Ford, G. (1983) Inequalities in old age: An examination of age, sex and class differences in a sample of community elderly, *Ageing and Society*, 3: 184–208.

Thane, P. (1978) The muddled history of retiring at 60 and 65, *New Society*, 3 August, pp. 234–36.

Thomas, K. (1978) *Religion and the Decline of Magic*. London: Weidenfeld and Nicolson.

Tomlin, S. (1989) 'Abuse of elderly people – An unnecessary and preventable problem', British Geriatric Society, Occasional Paper, London: British Geriatric Society.

Townsend, P. (1957) *The Family Life of Old People*. London: Routledge and Kegan Paul.

Townsend, P. (1981) The structured dependency of the elderly: A creation of social policy in the twentieth century, *Ageing and Society*, 1(1): 5–28.

Tyler, M. and Abbott, P. (1994) 'The commodification of sexuality: Sexualized labour markets', paper presented to Conference on Work, Employment and Society in the 1990s: Changing Boundaries, Changing Experiences, University of Kent, Canterbury, 12–14 September.

Ungerson, C. (1983) Why do women care? In J. Finch and D. Groves (eds) *A Labour of Love: Women, Work and Caring*. London: Routledge and Kegan Paul.

Ungerson, C. (1987) *Policy is Personal: Gender and Informal Care*. London: Tavistock.

Ve, H. (1984) Women's mutual alliances: Altruism as a basis for interaction. In H. Holter (ed.) *Patriarchy in a Welfare Society*. Bergen: University of Bergen.

Vincent, J. and Mucrovĉić, Ž. (1993) Lifestyles and perceptions of elderly people and old age in Bosnia and Hercegovina. In S. Arber and M. Evandrou (eds) *Ageing, Independence and the Life Course*. London: Jessica Kingsley Publishers.

Vonhof, T. (1991) 'Homemaker services to the elderly: Impact on family caregivers', unpublished MSc thesis. Department of Family Studies, University of Guelph, Ontario, Canada.

Waerness, K. (1987) The rationality of care. In A. Sassoon (ed.) *Women and the State*. London: Hutchinson.

Walby, S. (1986) *Patriarchy at Work*. Oxford: Polity Press.

Walby, S. (1994) Is citizenship gendered? *Sociology*, 28(2): 379–95.

Walker, A. (1980) The social creation of poverty and dependency in old age, *Journal of Social Policy*, 9(1): 49–75.

Walker, A. (1981) Towards a political economy of old age, *Ageing and Society*, 1(1): 73–94.

Walker, A. (ed.) (1982) *Community Care: The Family, the State and Social Policy*. Oxford: Blackwell.

Walker, A. (1987) The poor relation: Poverty among older women. In C. Glendinning and J. Millar (eds) *Women and Poverty in Britain*. Hemel Hempstead: Harvester Wheatsheaf.

Wall, R. (1992) Relationships between generations in British families past and present. In C. Marsh and S. Arber (eds) *Families and Households: Divisions and Change*. London: Macmillan.

Warren, D.I. (1981) *Helping Networks: How People Cope with Problems in the Urban Community*. Notre Dame, IN: University of Notre Dame.

Weiss, J. (1988) Family violence and research methodology and design. In L. Ohlin and M. Tonfry (eds) *Family Violence*. Chicago, IL: University of Chicago Press.

Wenger, G. C. (1980) *Mid-Wales: Deprivation or Development.* Cardiff: University of Wales Press.

Wenger, G. C. (1983) Loneliness: A problem of measurement. In D. Jerrome (ed.) *Ageing in Modern Society.* London: Croom Helm.

Wenger, G. C. (1984) *The Supportive Network: Coping with Old Age.* London: Allen and Unwin.

Wenger, G. C. (1986) A longitudinal study of changes and adaptations in the support networks of Welsh elderly over 75, *Journal of Cross-Cultural Gerontology,* 1(3): 277–304.

Wenger, G. C. (1987a) *Relationships in Old Age – Inside Support Networks,* research report. Bangor: Centre for Social Policy Research and Development, University of Wales.

Wenger, G. C. (1987b) Dependence, interdependence and reciprocity after 80, *Journal of Aging Studies,* 1(4): 355–77.

Wenger, G. C. (1990) Elderly carers: The need for appropriate intervenion, *Ageing and Society,* 10(2): 1–23.

Wenger, G. C. (1992a) Morale in old age: A review of the evidence, *International Journal of Geriatric Psychiatry,* 7: 699–708.

Wenger, G. C. (1992b) *Help in Old Age – Facing up to Change: A Longitudinal Network Study.* Liverpool: Liverpool University Press.

Wenger, G. C. (1994a) *Understanding Support Networks and Community Care.* Aldershot: Avebury.

Wenger, G. C. (1994b) *Support Networks of Older People: A Guide for Practitioners.* Bangor: Centre for Social Policy Research and Development, University of Wales.

Wenger, G. C. (1995) A comparison of urban with rural support networks: Liverpool and North Wales, *Ageing and Society* 15: 59–81.

Wenger, G. C. and Shahtamasebi, S. (1990) Variations in support networks: Some policy implications. In J. Mogey, P. Somlai and J. Trost (eds), *Aiding and Ageing: The Coming Crisis.* Westport, CT: Greenwood Press.

White, L. and Edwards, J. (1990) Emptying the nest and parental well-being: An analysis of national panel data, *American Sociological Review,* 55: 235–42.

Williams, R. (1990) *A Protestant Legacy: Attitudes to Death and Illness Among Older Aberdonians.* Oxford: Clarendon Press.

Wilson, E. (1975) *Women and the Welfare State.* London: Virago.

Wilson, G. (1987) Money: Patterns of responsibility and irresponsibility in marriage. In J. Brannen and G. Wilson (eds) *Give and Take in Families: Studies in Resource Distribution.* London: Allen and Unwin.

Wilson, G. (1994) Abuse of elderly men and women among clients of a community psychogeriatric service, *British Journal of Social Work,* 24(6): 681–700.

Wolf, R. (1988) Elder abuse: Ten years later, *Journal of the American Gerontological Society,* 36(8): 758–62.

Wolf, R. and Pillemer, K. (1989) *Helping Elderly Victims.* New York: Columbia University Press.

Wright, L. (1991) The impact of Alzheimer's disease on the marital relationship, *Gerontologist,* 31: 224–37.

Young, M. and Willmott, P. (1973) *The Symmetrical Family.* London: Routledge and Kegan Paul.

Young, M. and Schuller, T. (1991) *Life After Work.* London: Harper Collins.

Zarb, G. (1993) 'Forgotten but not gone'. The experience of ageing with a disability. In S.

Arber and M. Evandrou (eds) *Ageing, Independence and the Life Course.* London: Jessica Kingsley Publishers.

Zarit, S., Todd, P. and Zarit, J. (1986) Subjective burden of husbands and wives as caregivers: A longitudinal study, *The Gerontologist,* 26(3): 260–66.

INDEX

Abbott, P., 3, 37, 59
Abdela, L., 57
Abrams, M., 117–18, 165
Abrams, P., 115
Abrams, S., 115
Abu-Laban, S., 31
abuse, 96, 144–57, 177
    and carer stress, 144–5, 147–52,
        154–7, 159
    and family violence, 27, 144, 146,
        148–50, 157
    and gender, 38, 144–5, 147–8, 150–2
    and power, 144, 149, 151–7
accounts, 37, 42–3, 94, 103, 118–19, 121,
    124–5, 127, 151
Acker, J., 4, 30, 34, 38–41
active life expectancy, 163, 174
activities of daily living, 11, 130, 133
    instrumental, 133
Adams, K., 25
Ade-Ridder, L., 89
adjustment, 17–18, 52, 57, 65, 67
advocacy, 153
affinity theories, 71–2
age
    adding on, 32–4, 36

advanced old, 10–11, 98–100, 102–13,
    132, 163
barriers/boundaries/restrictions, 23,
    26–7, 53, 62, 71
chronological, 5–8, 10, 13, 21–3, 26,
    98–9, 174
discrimination, see discrimination
differential in marriage, see marital
meanings of, 2, 5, 7, 10, 13, 24, 173–4
middle, see middle-age
norms, see norms
physiological, 5–6, 10–11, 13, 27, 99,
    117, 120, 174
of retirement, see retirement
social, 5, 7–8, 12–13, 158
as a variable, 2, 30–1, 34–5
ageism, 2, 6–7, 99, 156, 174, 178
    see also stereotypes
agency, 4, 5, 16, 19–21, 28–9, 115, 155
    collective, 36, 40
    human, 5, 20, 29, 41
Ages of Man, 21, 24
alcohol/drugs, 149
Allatt, P., 3, 55, 114
Alzheimer's disease, 27, 121, 124, 126–7
    see also dementia